We dedicate this book to all the children, and youth, along with their families and loved ones, who are bravely navigating a bone marrow transplant, and to all the courageous providers who care for them.

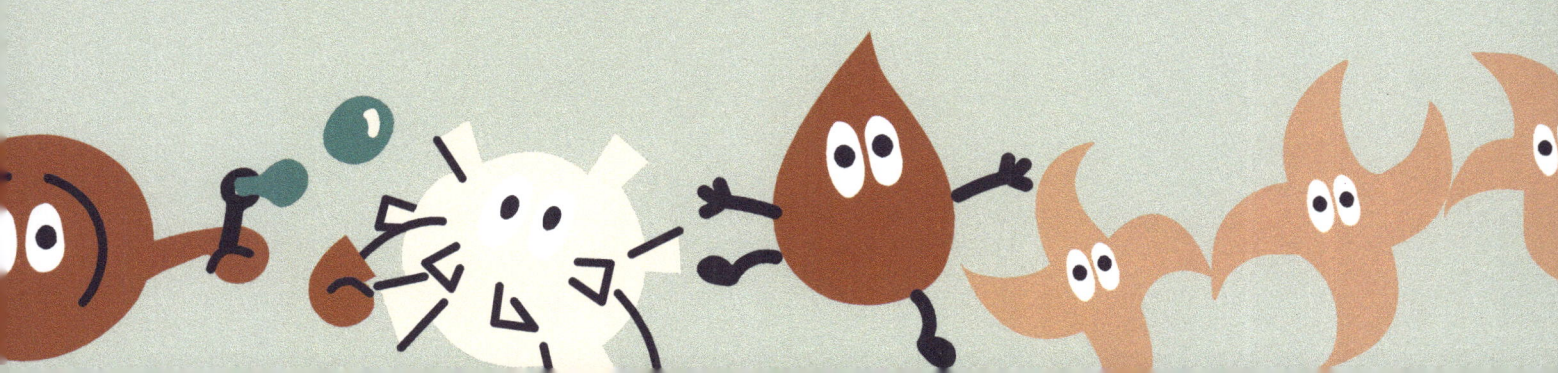

Text copyright © 2023 Child Core Family Support LLC.

All rights reserved.

No part of this book may be reproduced or transmitted in any form or by any means, electronic or mechanical, including photocopying, recording, or by any information storage and retrieval system, without written permission from the publisher.

The only exception is brief quotations for reviews.

For information please contact author at hello@childcorefamilysupport.com

ISBN: 979-8-9987553-1-6

The information in this book is based on our own education, research, and experience. It is designed to be used as a tool to support a child's understanding of the topic of a bone marrow transplant and not in lieu of already existing supports, consults, or medical information provided by Child Life Specialists or other medical professionals.

For more information about Child Life Specialists
and how they can help, go to childcorefamilysupport.com.

Written + Illustrated by Adrienne O'Connor, MS, CCLS
Written by Caitlin McNamara, MS, CCLS, CIMI

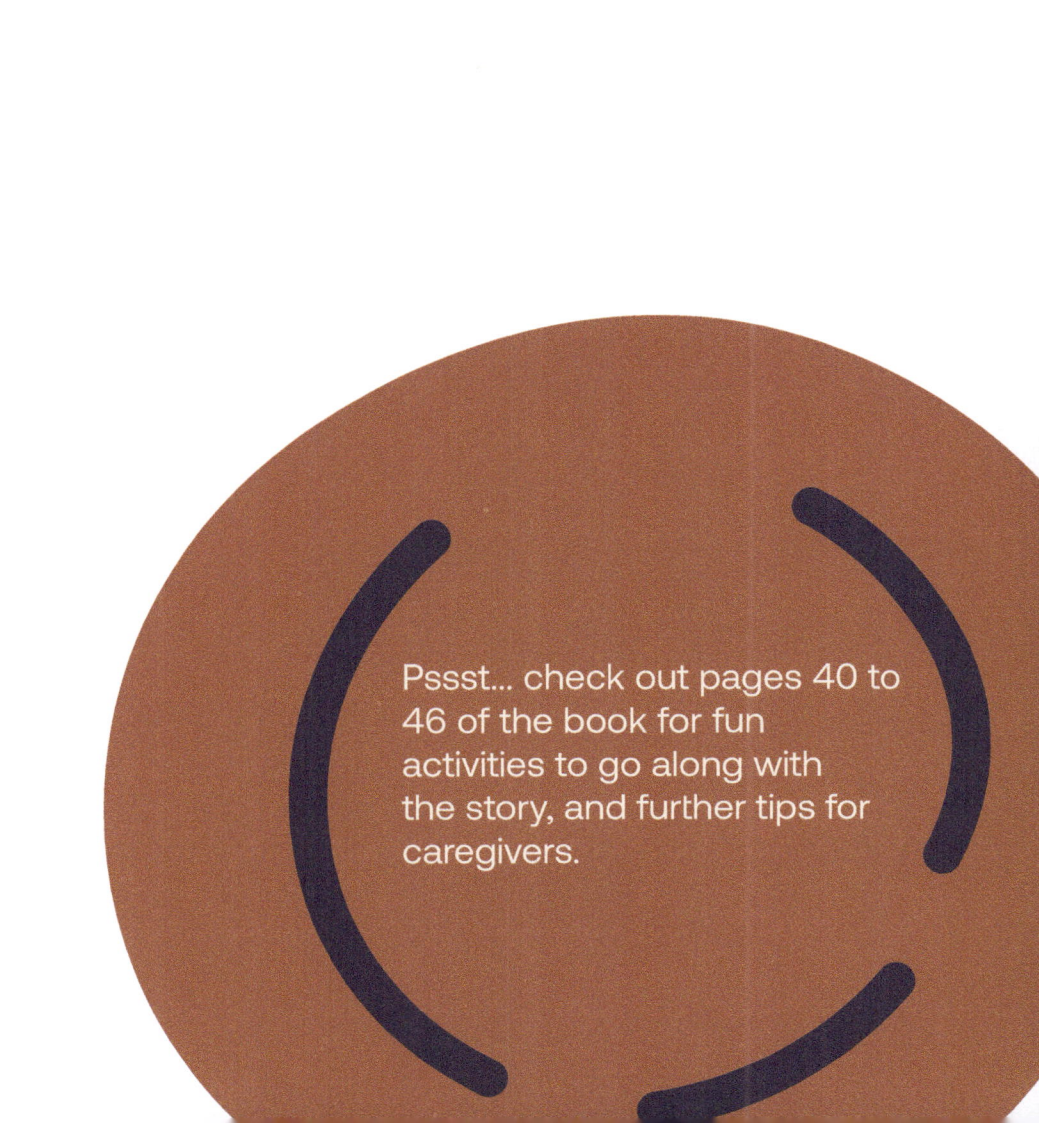

Pssst... check out pages 40 to 46 of the book for fun activities to go along with the story, and further tips for caregivers.

Have you ever heard adults use words you don't understand, and it makes you feel confused or curious to learn more?

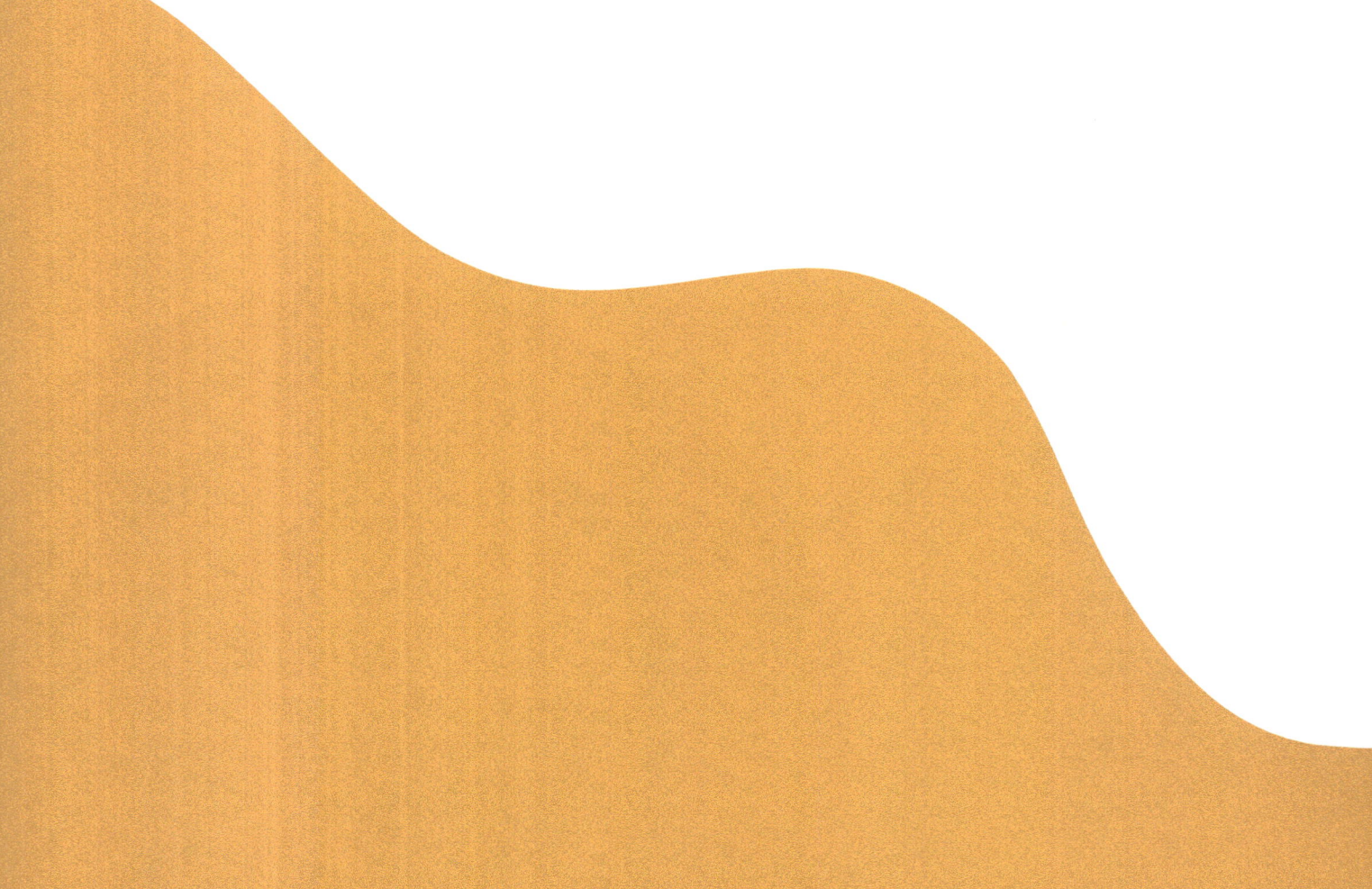

Well, this happened to me when I heard people using the words 'bone marrow' and 'bone marrow transplant'.

I finally asked what those words mean, and wow, did I learn a lot. Now, I want to share what I learned with you!

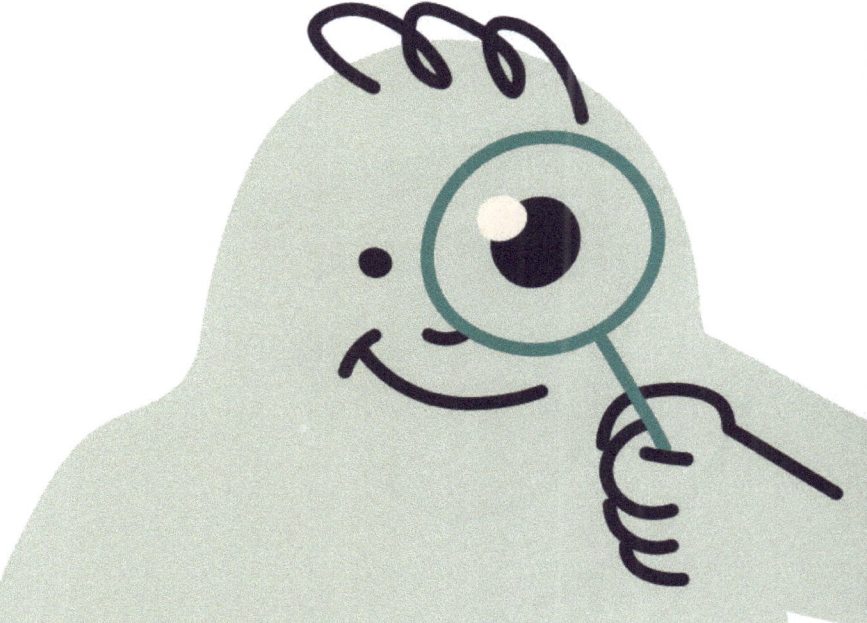

So you know what
a bone is, right?

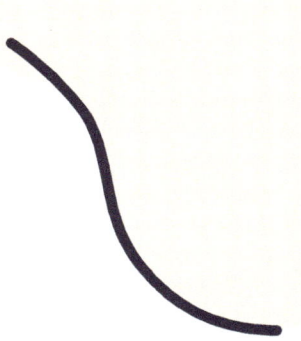

But have you heard the word
bone marrow?

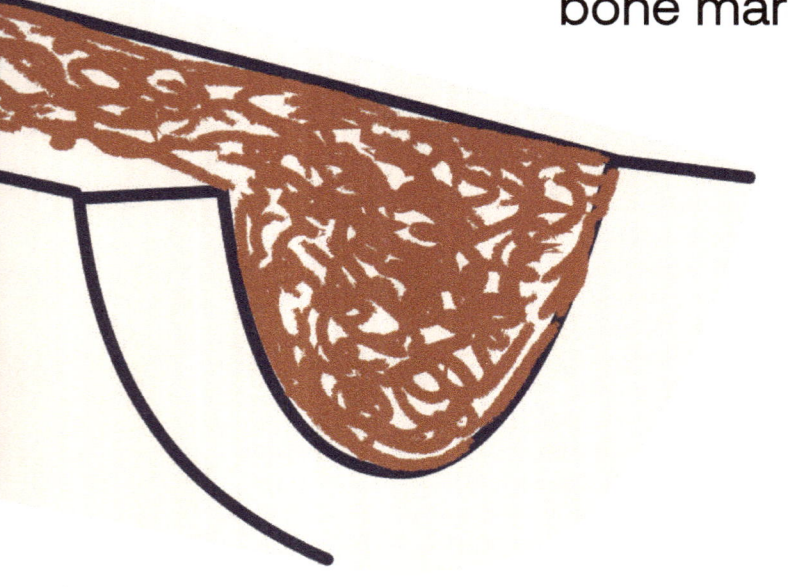

What about bone marrow
transplant?

Okay, okay, this could get confusing,
so let me start at the beginning....

...and talk about
how the body works.

The inside of our bodies are made up of different systems that all work together.

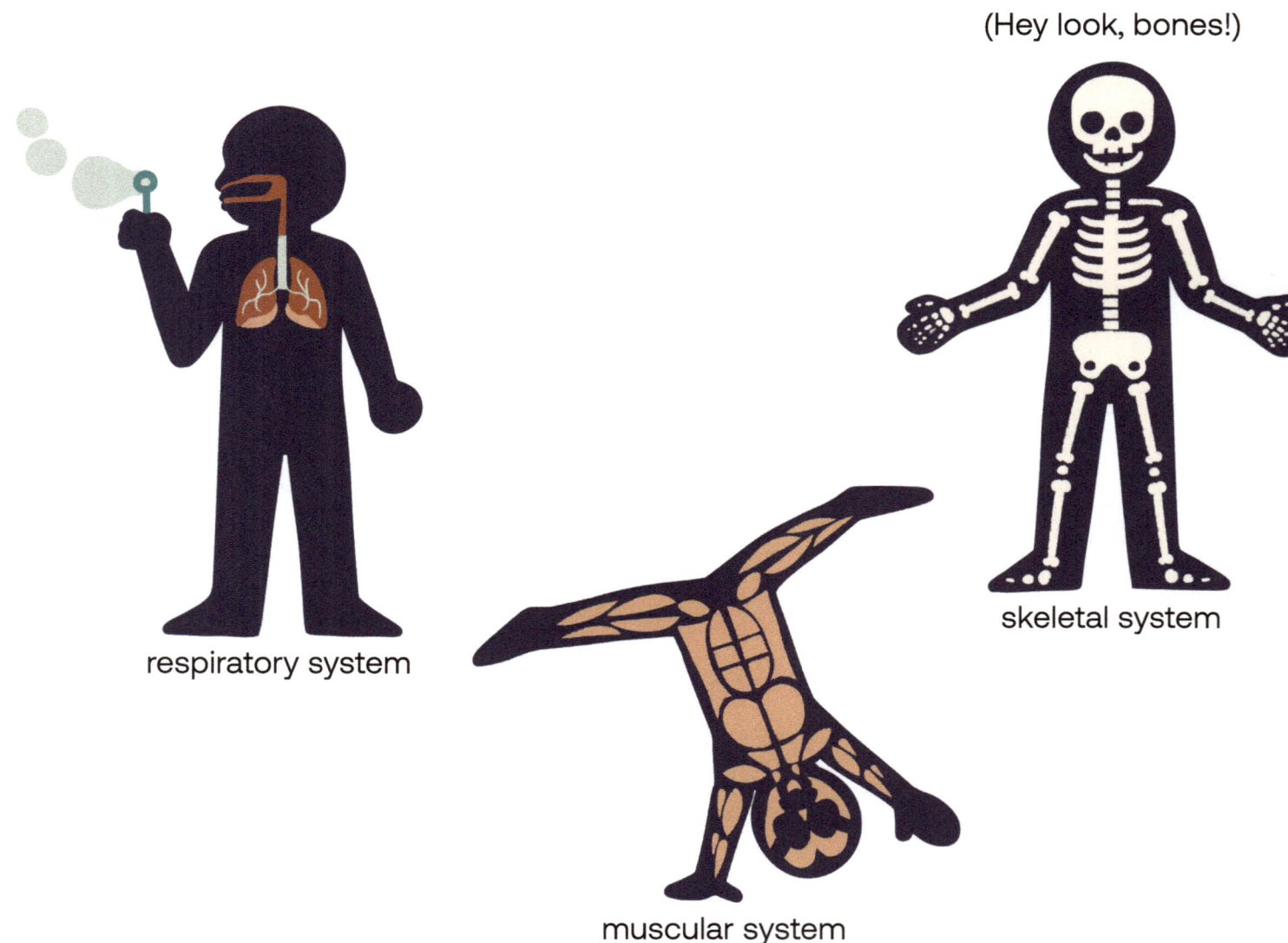

respiratory system

muscular system

(Hey look, bones!)

skeletal system

All of these systems have different jobs,

and they work together so we can do fun things like run, play, eat, think, and even blow bubbles!

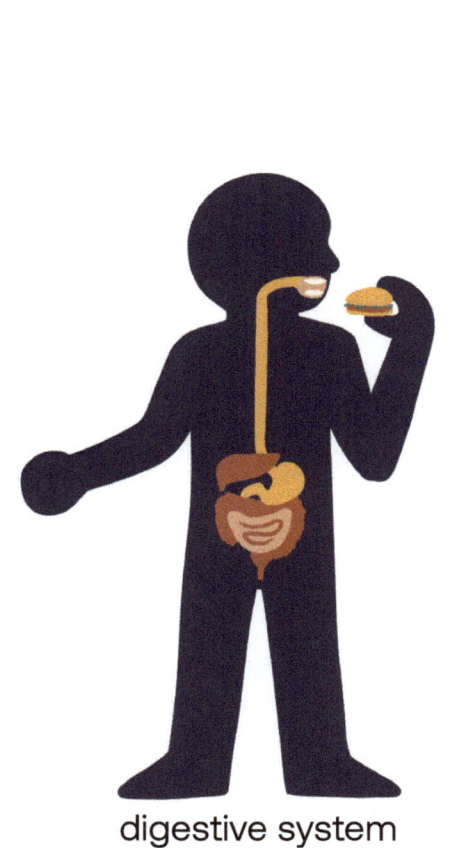
digestive system

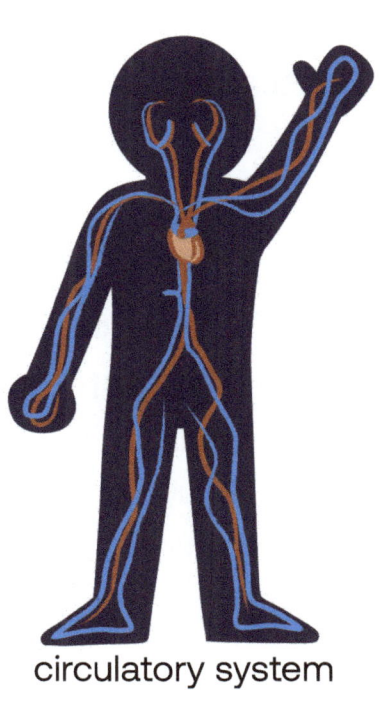
circulatory system

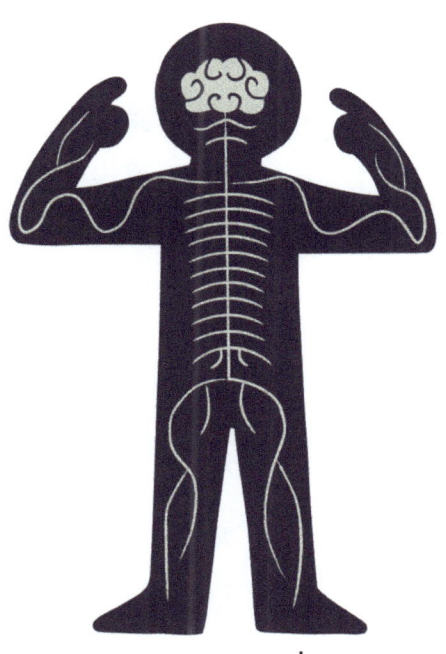
nervous system

Sometimes our body needs extra help, which is one reason why we might visit a doctor.

Like, if someone falls and breaks a bone in their arm, the doctor puts a cast on to help the bone heal.

Or if someone has a cough, the doctor gives them medicine to help their lungs feel better.

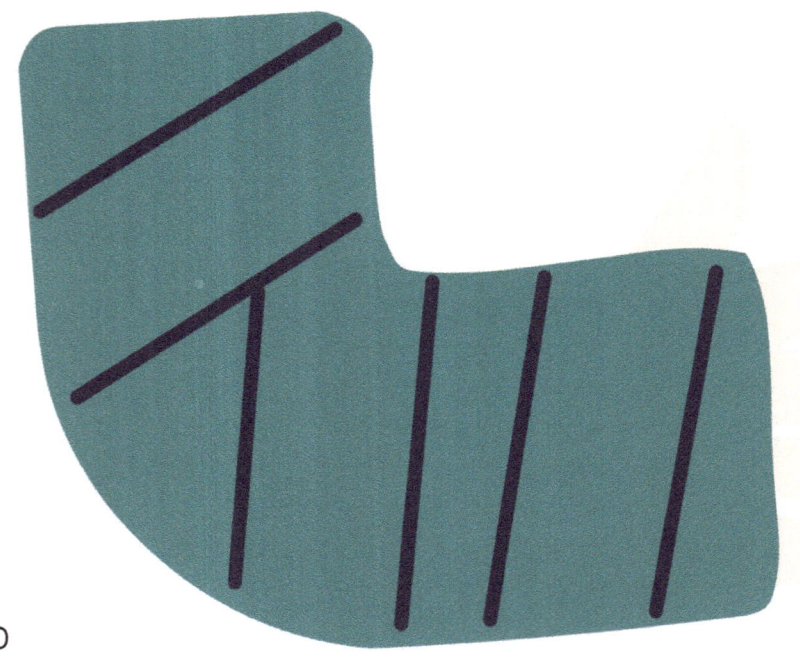

Another way a doctor takes care of someone's body is to help them make new blood.

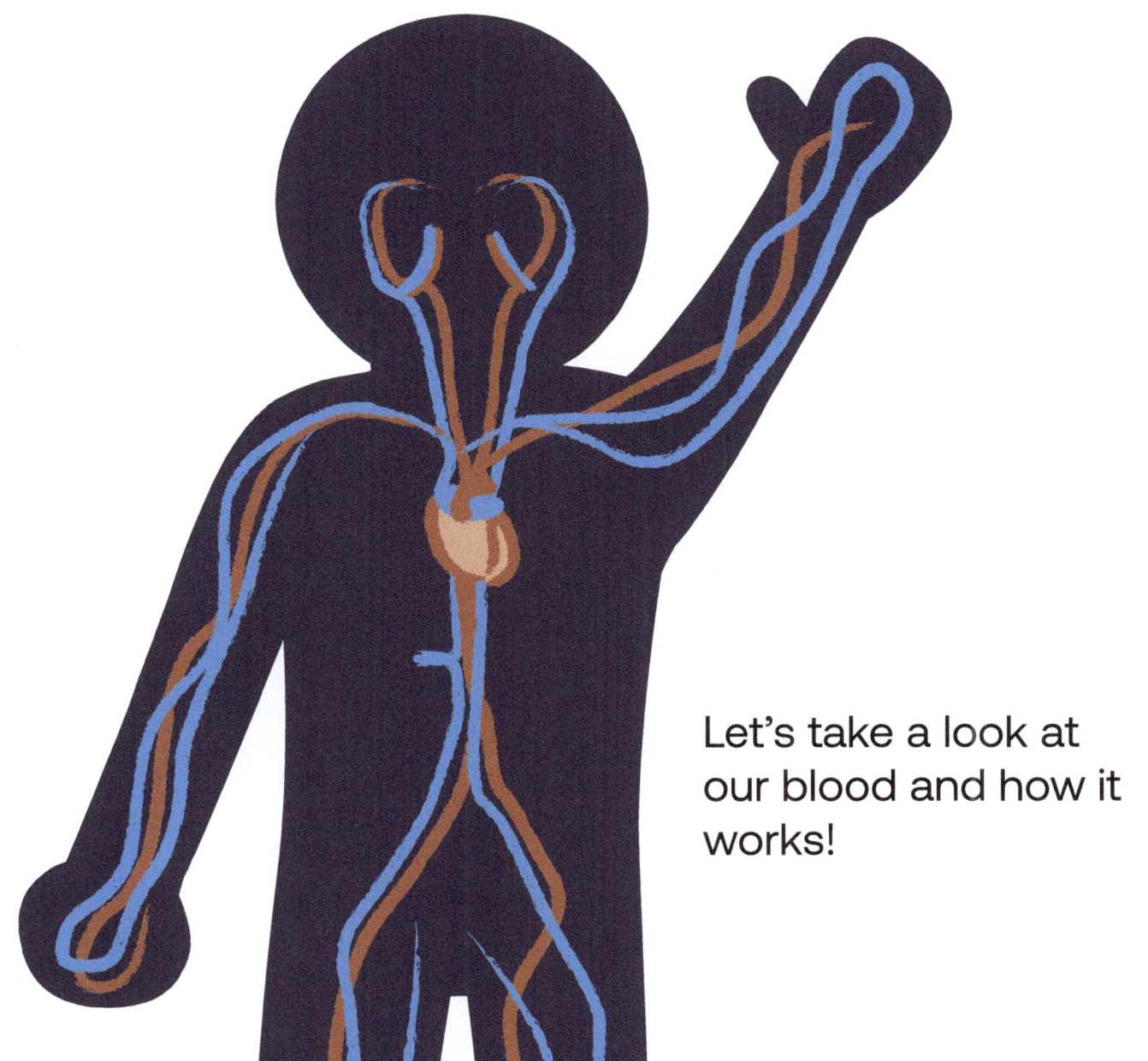

Let's take a look at our blood and how it works!

Blood is made up of tiny things called blood cells. There are 3 types of blood cells, and they all have different jobs to help our bodies.

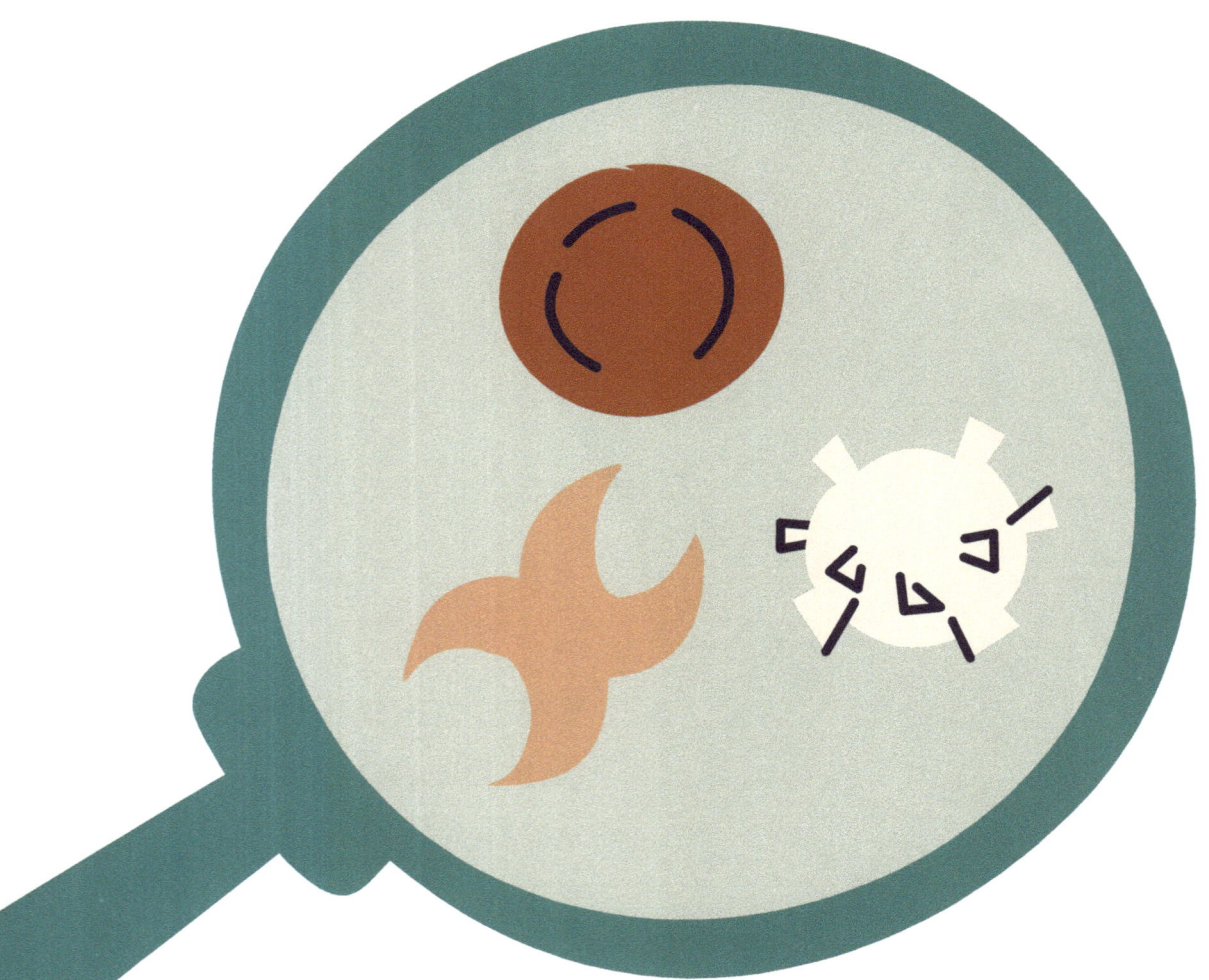

Let's see what they are!

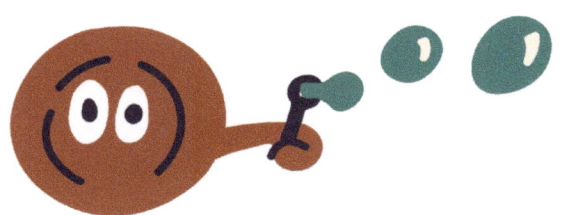
Red Blood Cells carry oxygen and healthy items like vitamins throughout our body and give us energy.

White Blood Cells help to protect us by fighting germs and infections.
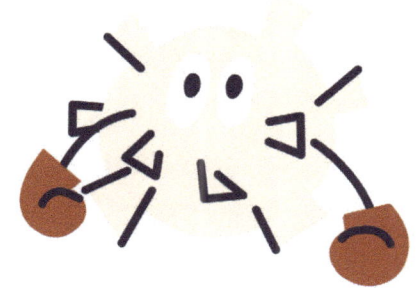

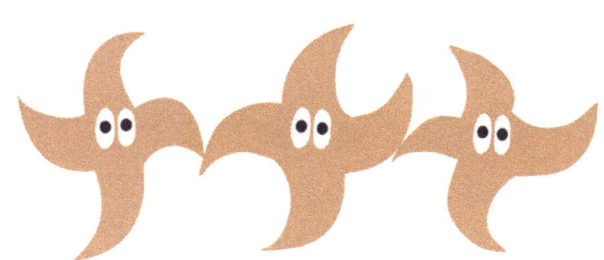
Platelets help our body heal, like when you get a cut or a bruise, your platelets clump together to form a seal, or scab, to stop the bleeding.

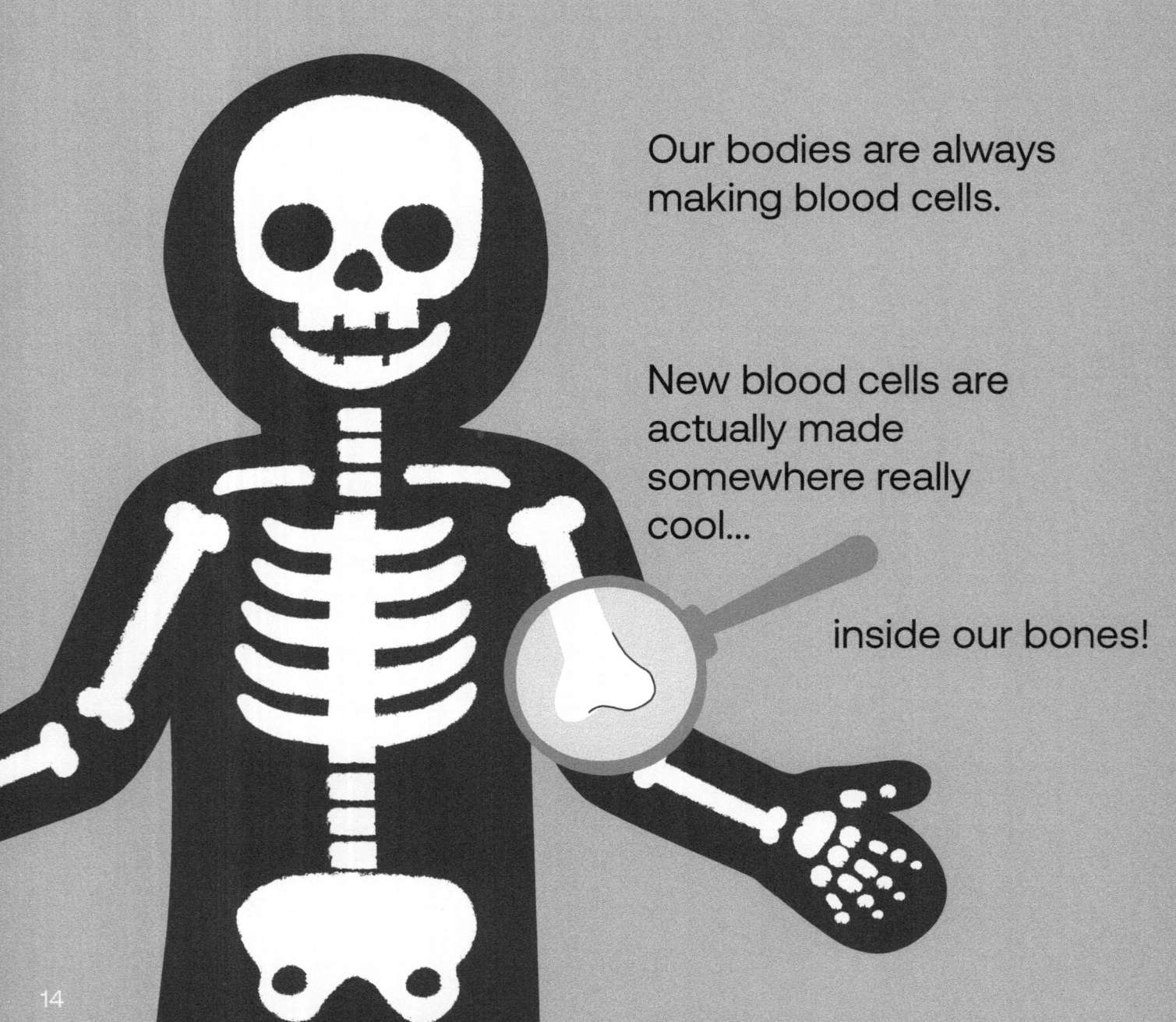

Our bodies are always making blood cells.

New blood cells are actually made somewhere really cool...

inside our bones!

The inside, squishy part of our bones is called

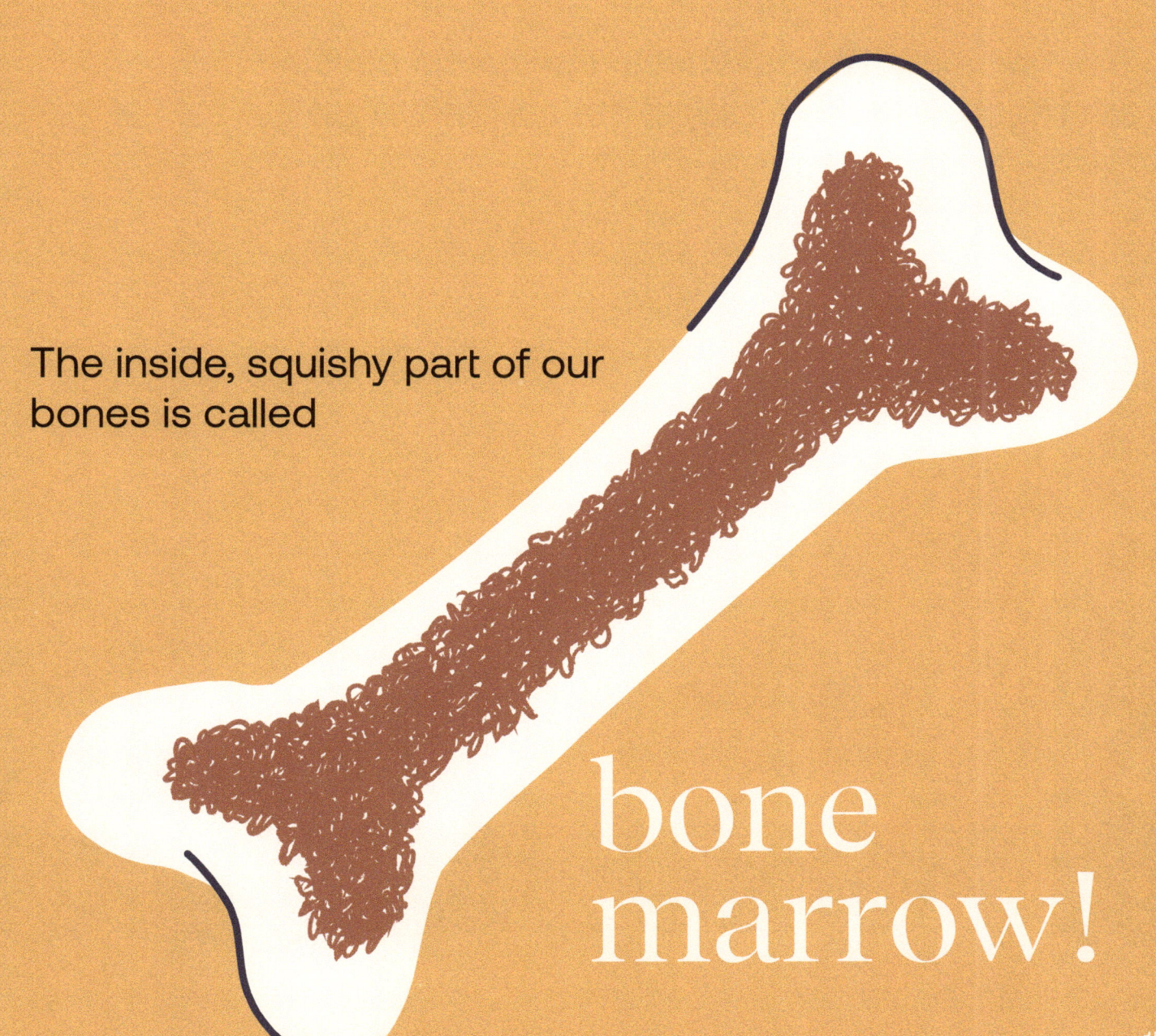

bone marrow!

The bone marrow is where new blood cells are made. It is like a blood making factory.

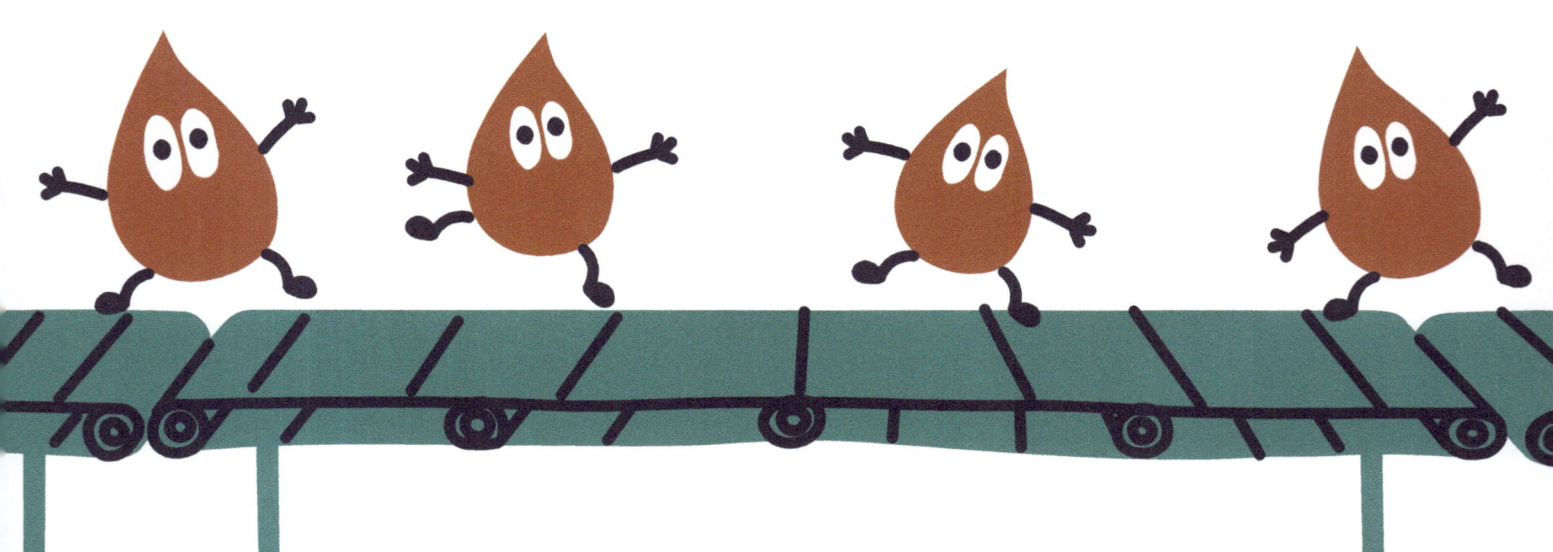

Here is a closer look at bone marrow.
It is where baby blood cells
grow into adult blood cells.

(baby blood cells are
also called stem cells)

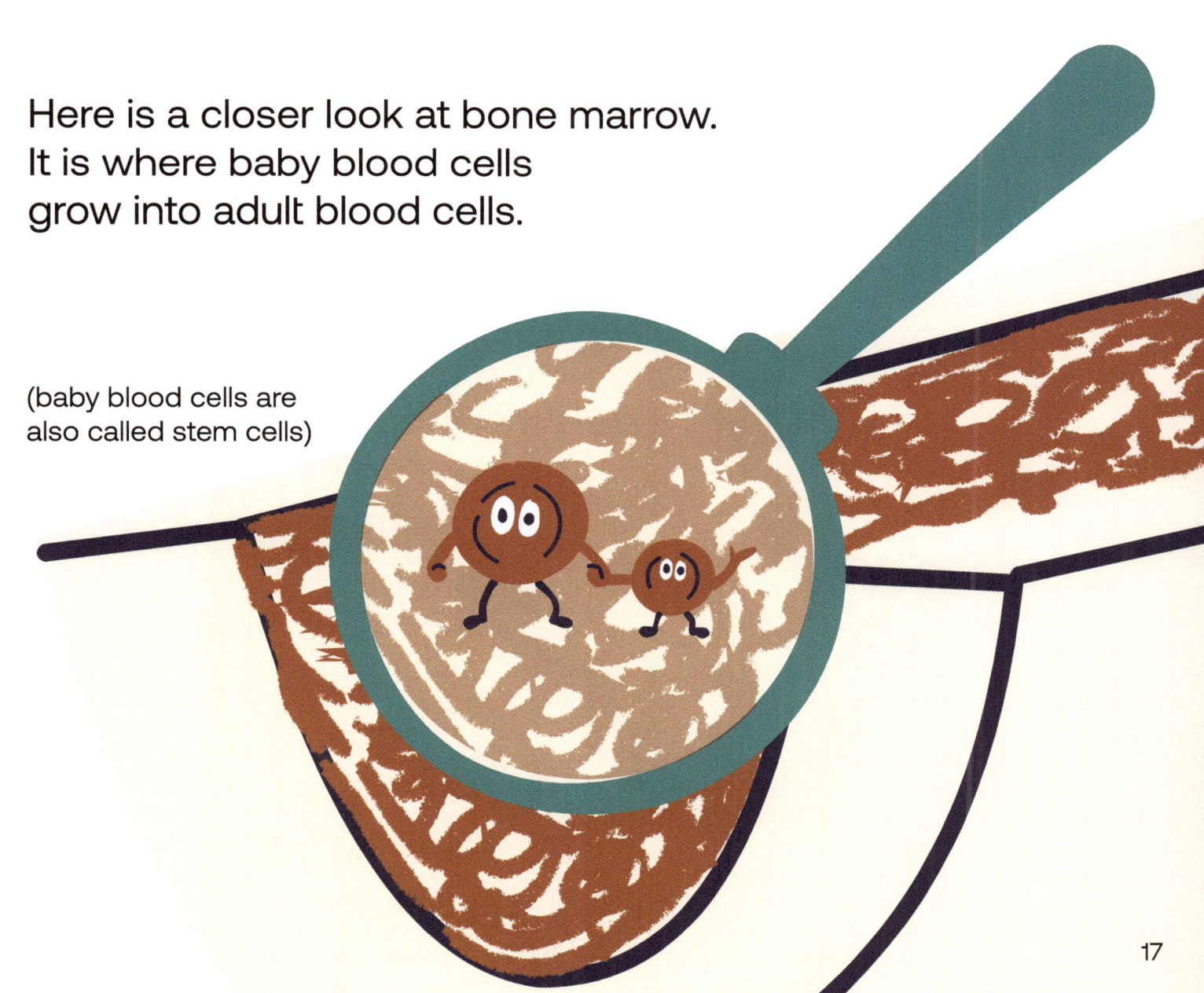

So, remember we talked about how doctors help our body?

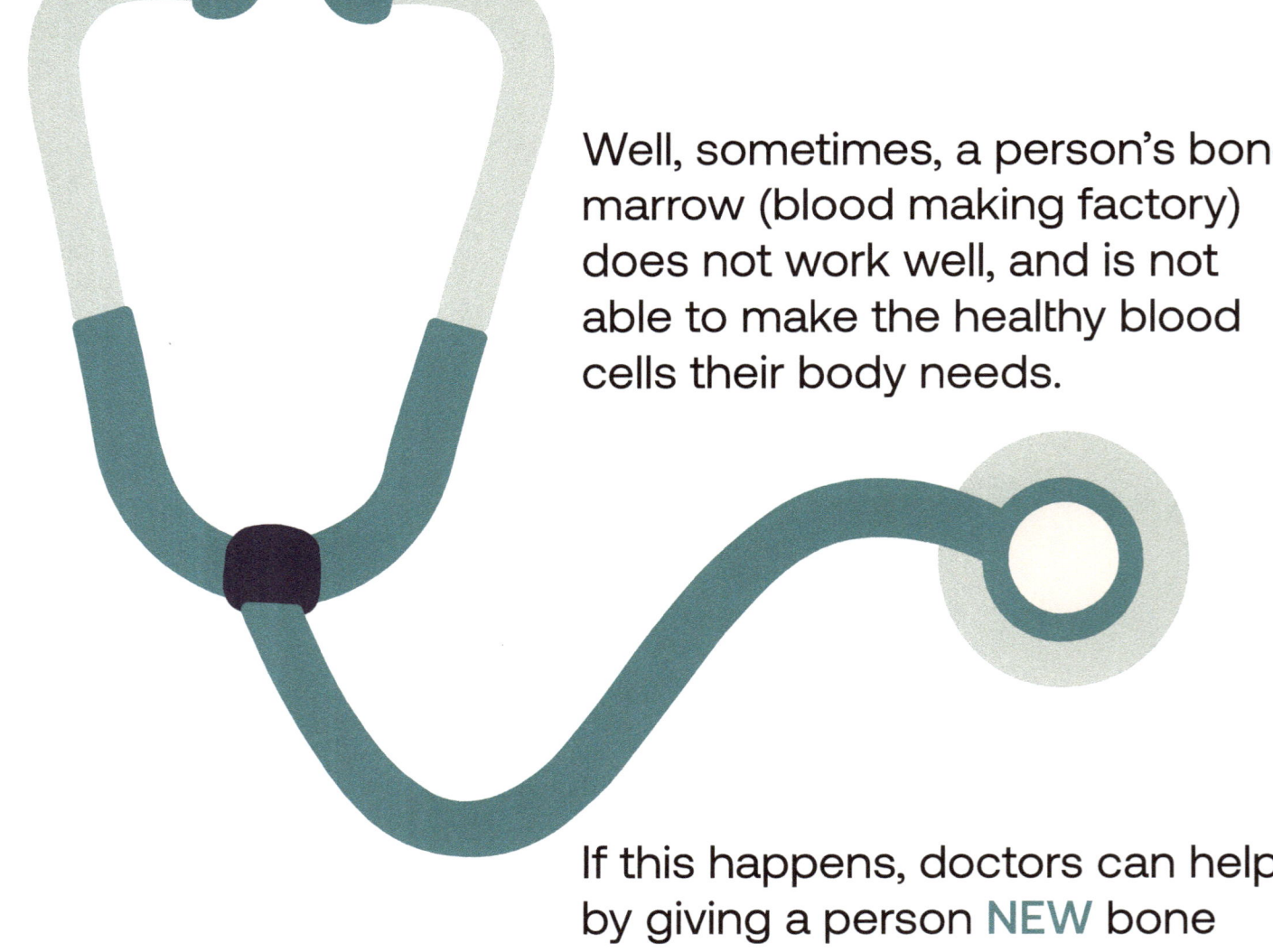

Well, sometimes, a person's bone marrow (blood making factory) does not work well, and is not able to make the healthy blood cells their body needs.

If this happens, doctors can help by giving a person NEW bone marrow!

What?! People can get new bone marrow?
Yup! This is called a BONE MARROW TRANSPLANT.

Transplant means getting something new, so a bone marrow transplant means getting NEW bone marrow!

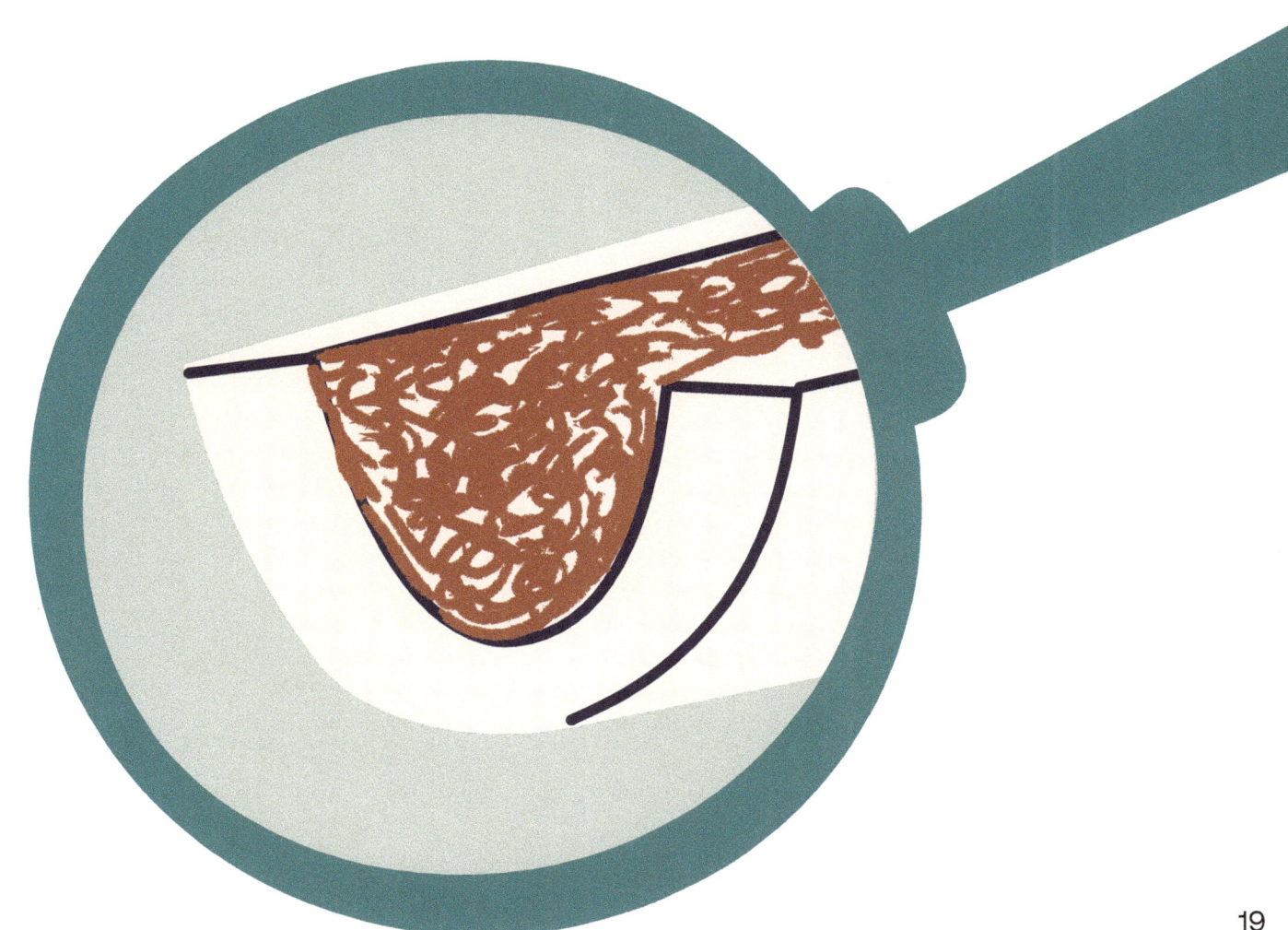

There are actually two steps to a bone marrow transplant.

First, medicine.

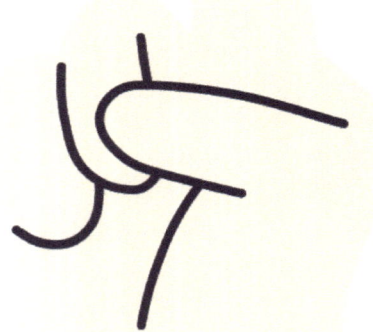

Second, the transplant.

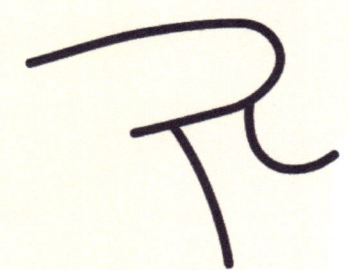

The first step is to get chemotherapy medicine. It is called "chemo" for short.

The chemo is very strong medicine whose job is like an eraser.

It erases the bone marrow to make room for the new, healthy bone marrow.

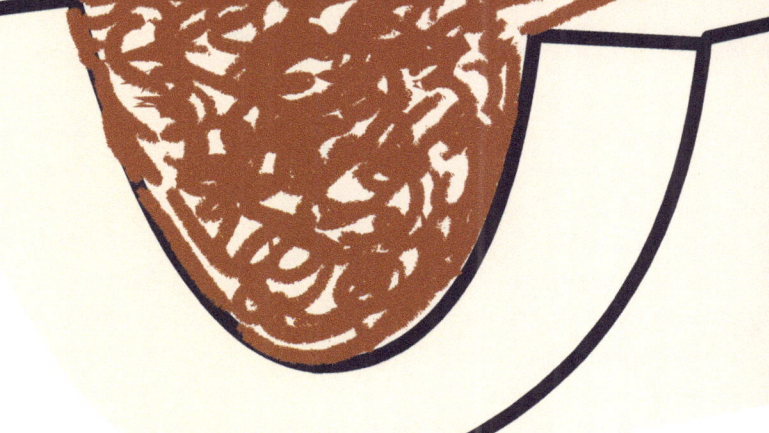

The second step is to get the new bone marrow.

A person gets the new, healthy bone marrow through a tube that is connected to their body.

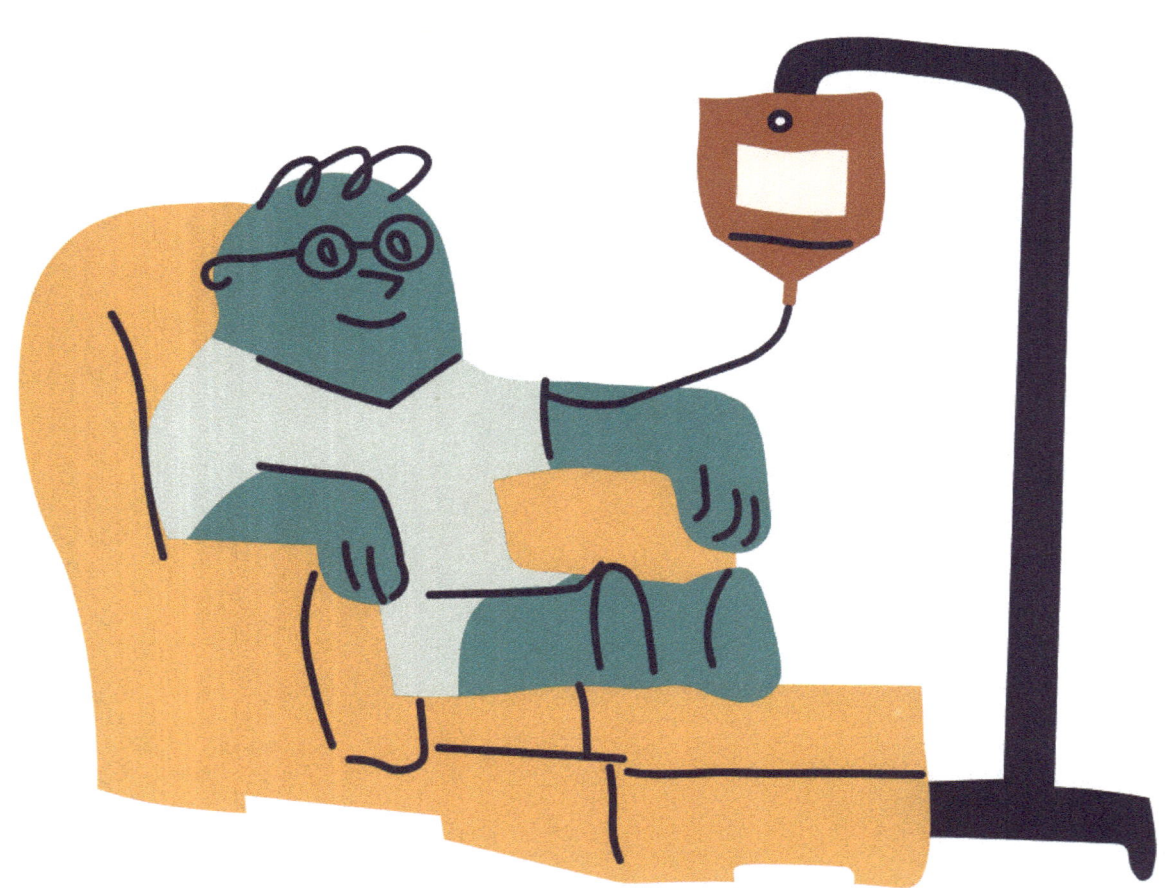

The new bone marrow will go through the tube into their body, travel into the middle part of their bones, and start growing new, healthy blood cells.

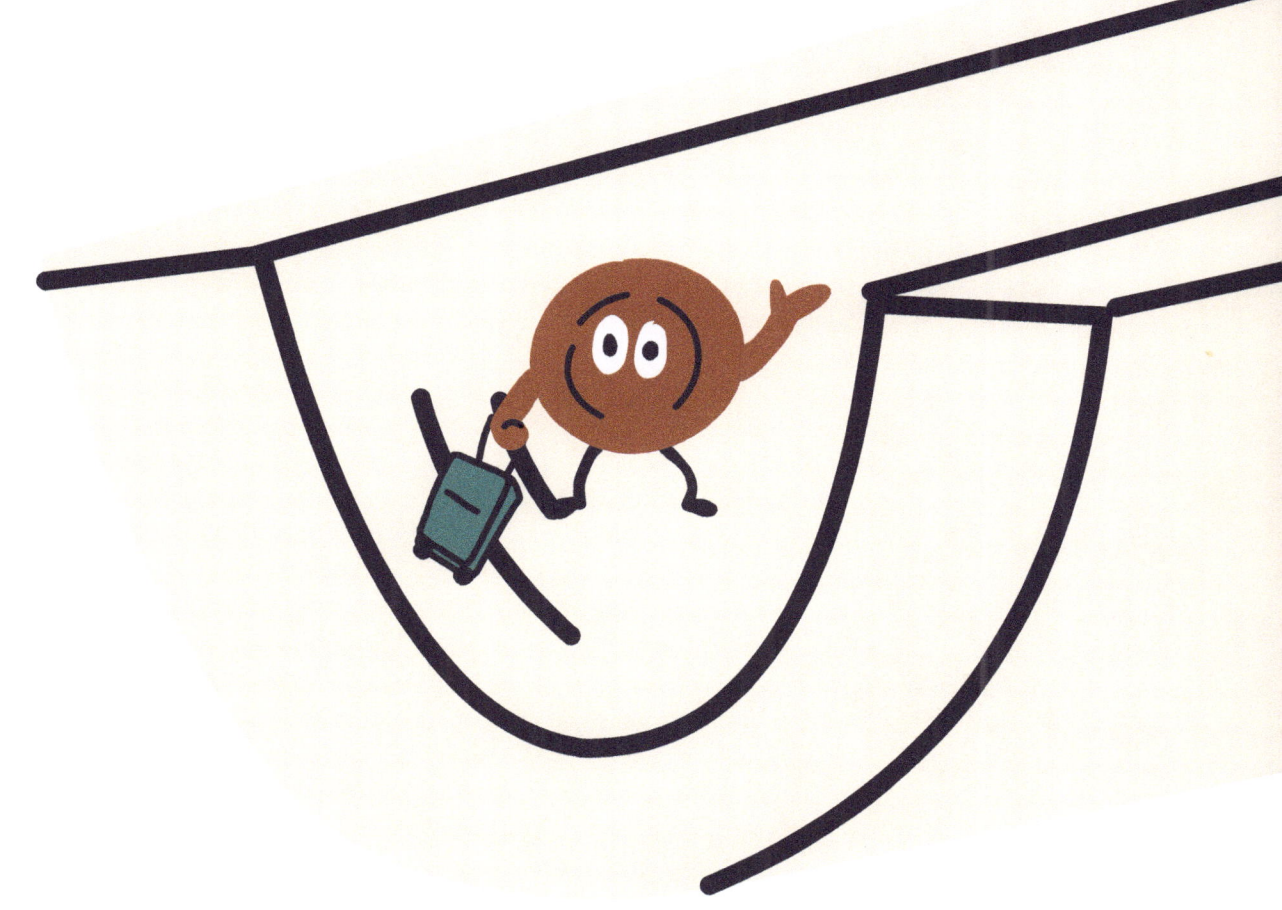

But wait, where does the new bone marrow come from?

The bone marrow can come from a person's own body, from their family member, or from someone they don't even know.

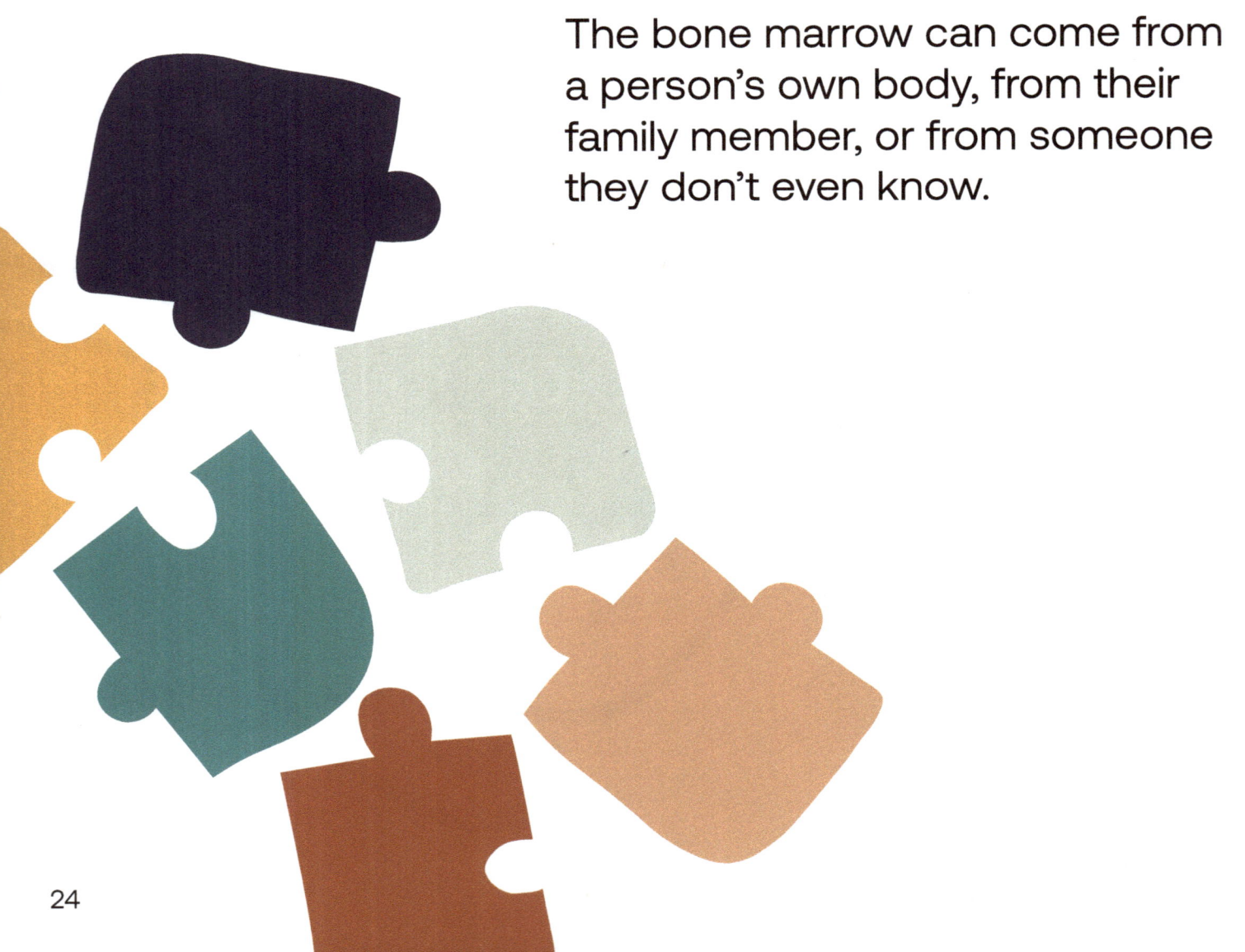

Everyone's bone marrow, or blood making factory, is different…

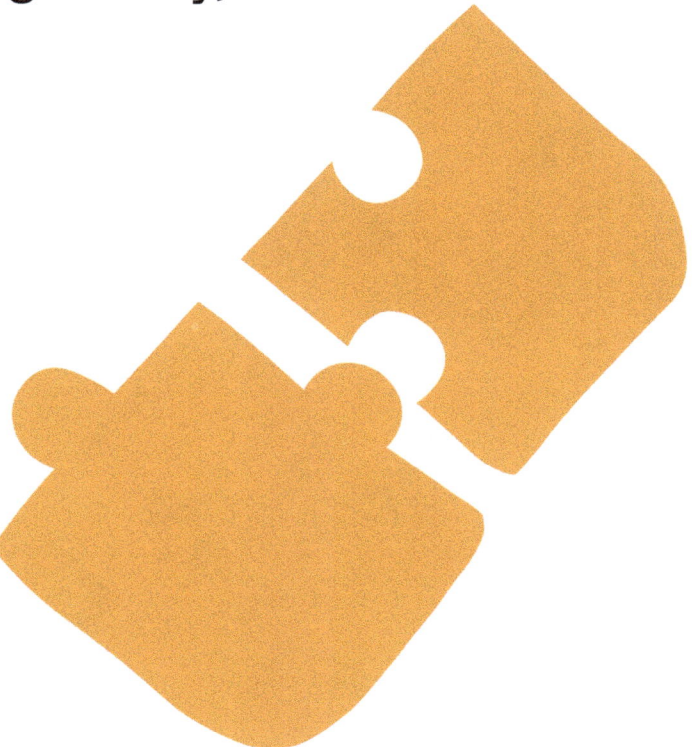

…so doctors do tests to search for the best match.

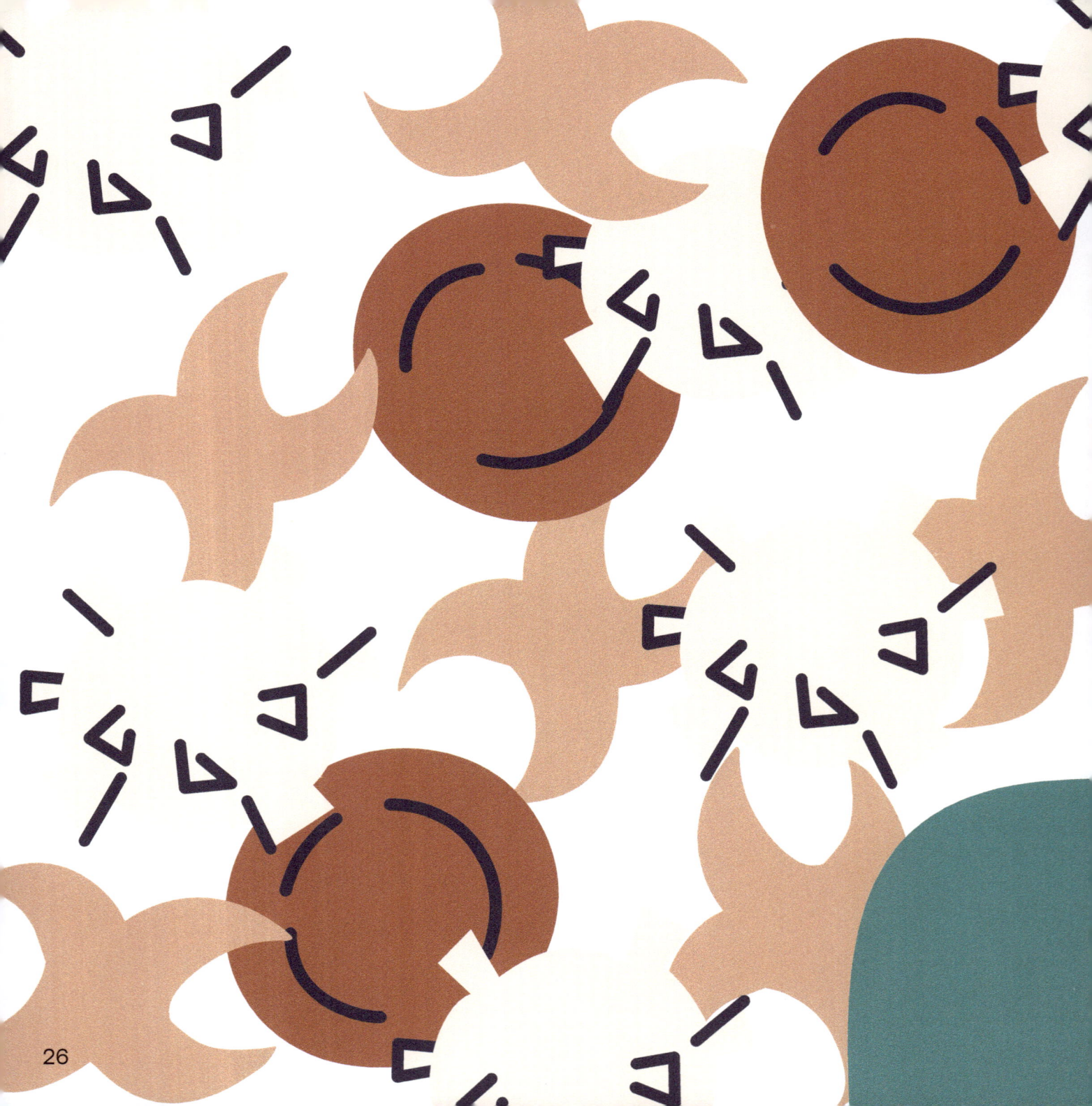

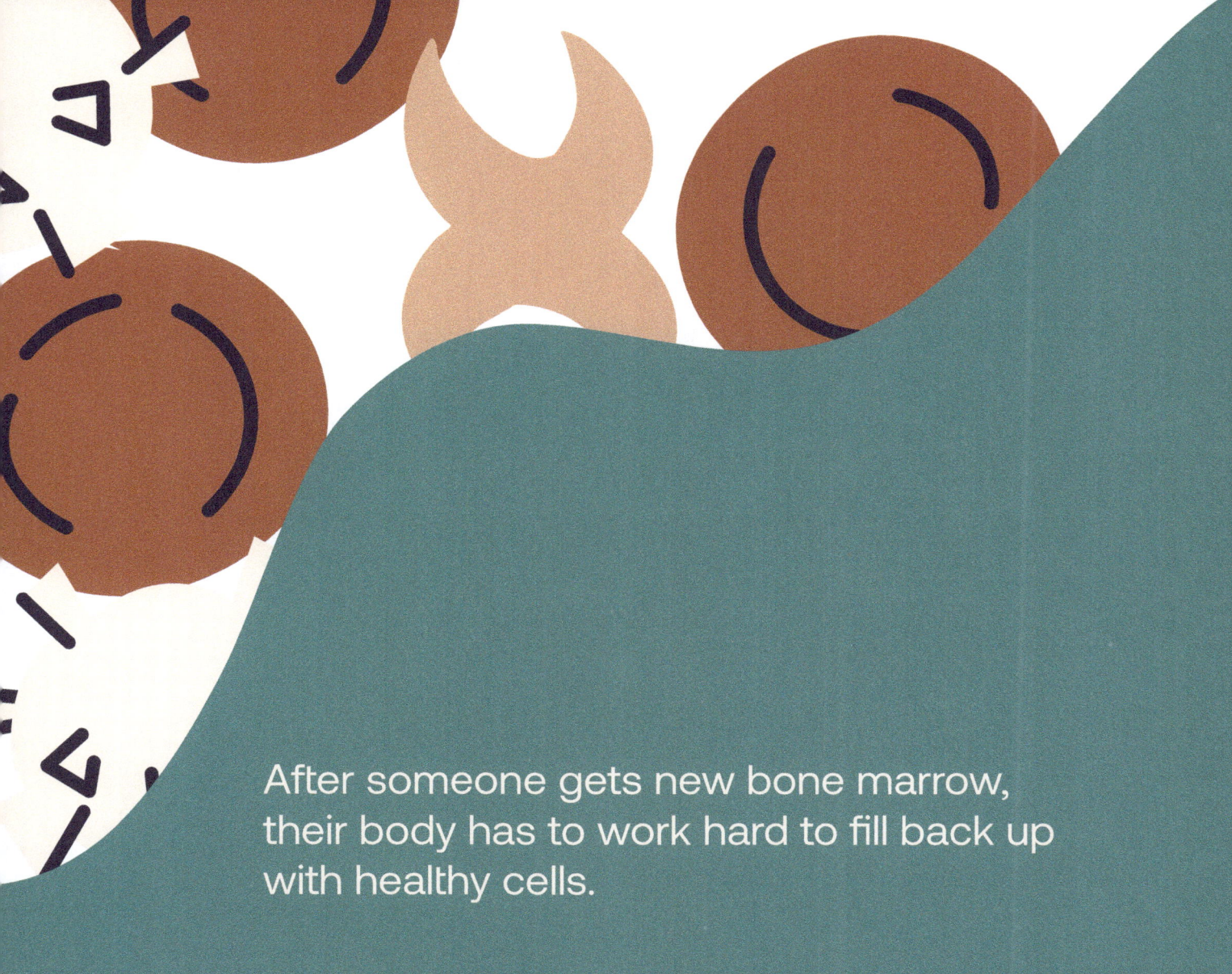

After someone gets new bone marrow, their body has to work hard to fill back up with healthy cells.

While their body is working hard to do this, they will spend some time in the hospital.

To help keep someone's body extra safe while the new, healthy blood cells are growing...

they may need to stay in their room and rest,

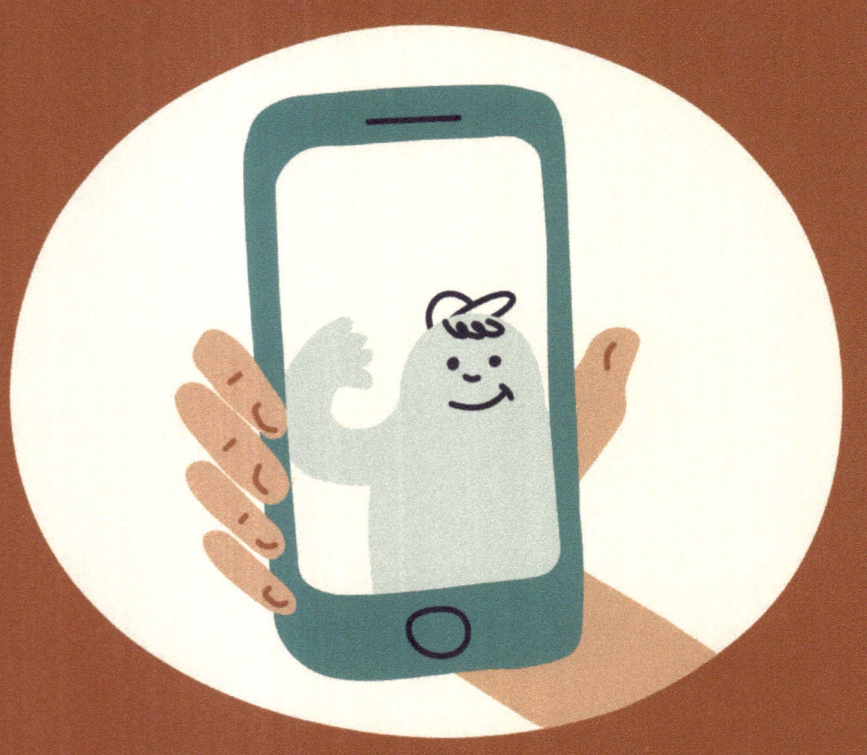

they might need to be careful about what they eat and drink,

kids might not be able to visit...

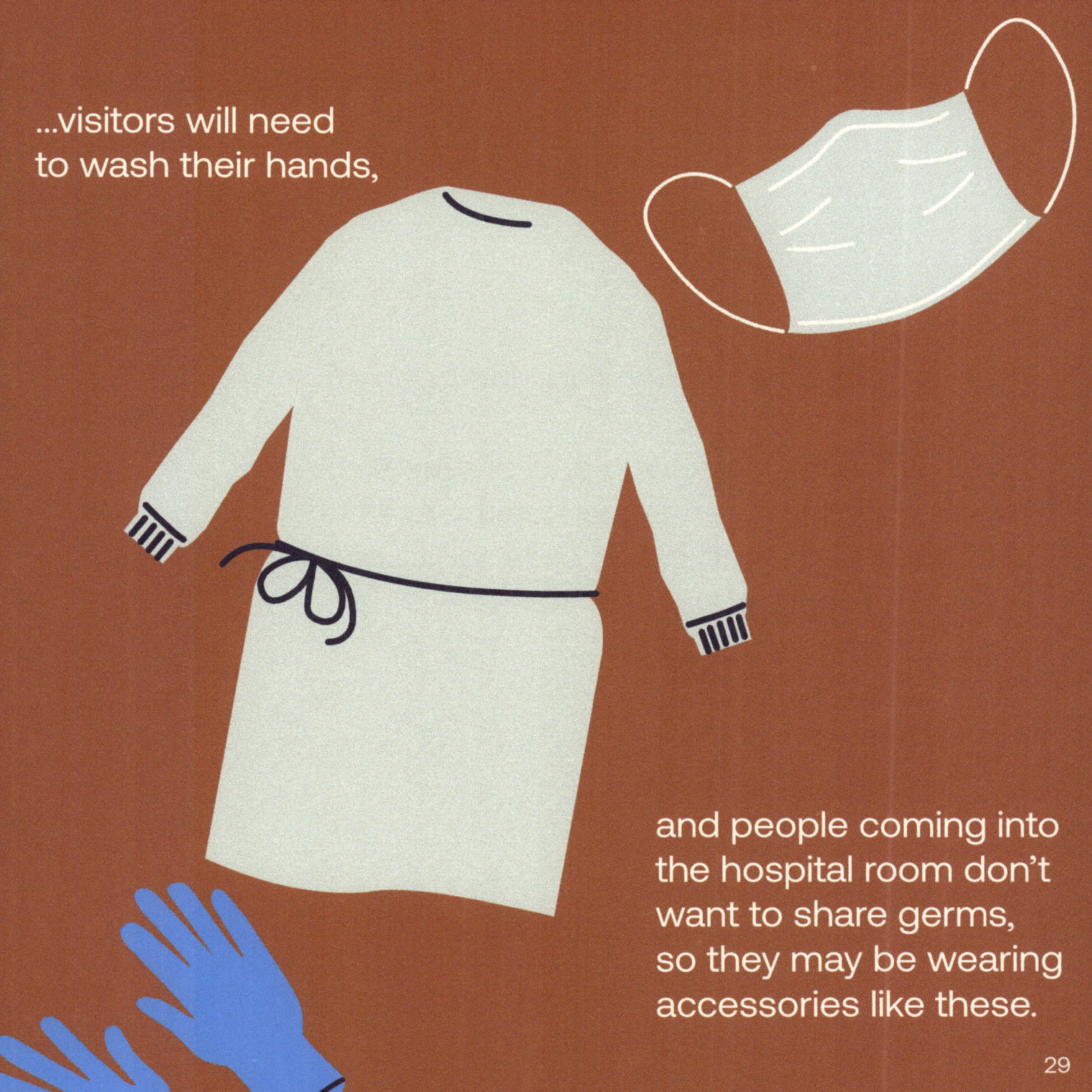

...visitors will need to wash their hands, and people coming into the hospital room don't want to share germs, so they may be wearing accessories like these.

Remember that strong medicine chemo?

Well, since it is so strong and erases the bone marrow, it can erase healthy cells too (remember the red blood cells, white blood cells, and platelets).

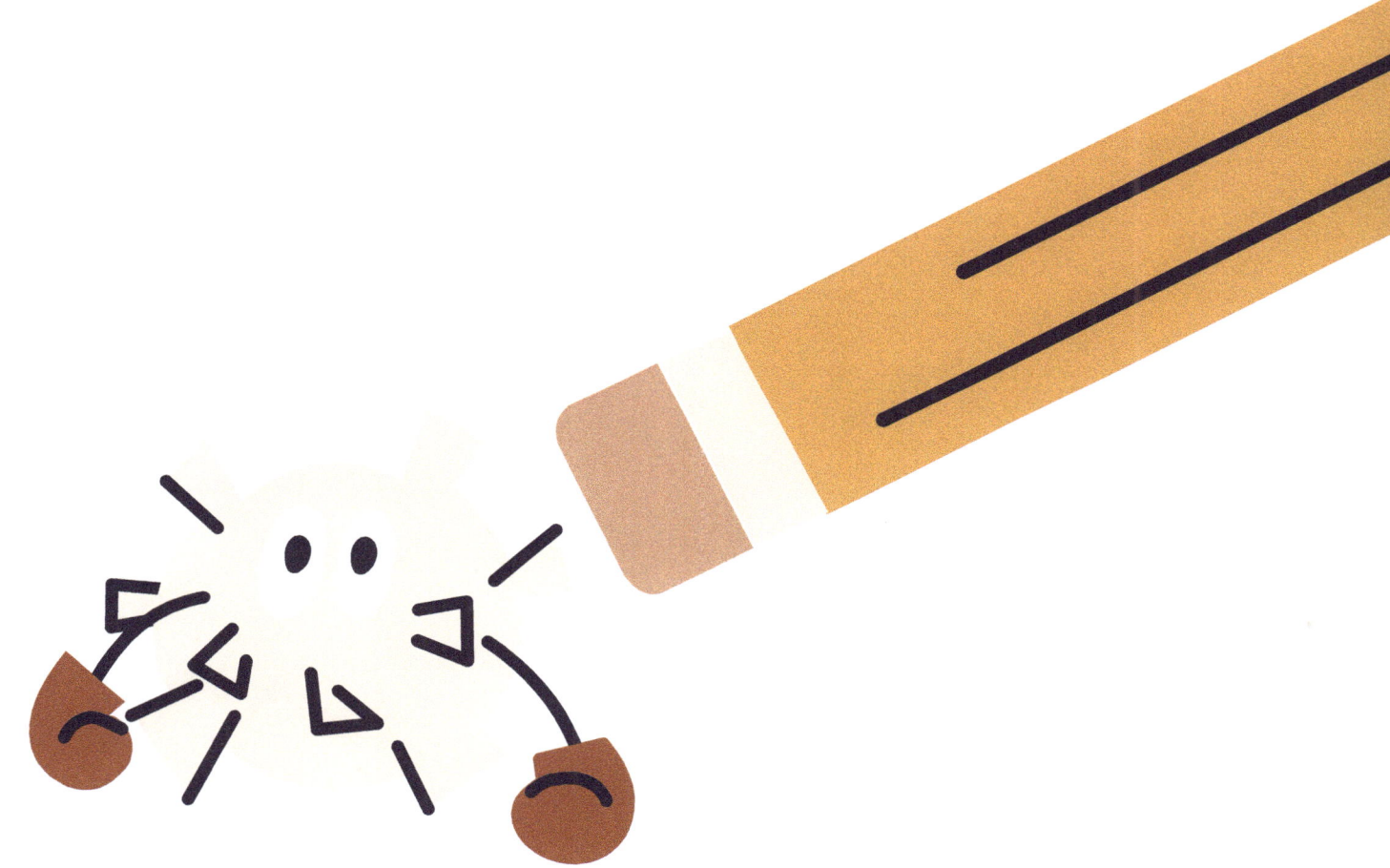

This is why it is important to be safe around germs, or why someone might not be feeling like doing the activities they usually like to do.

While someone is getting chemo medicine their body can look or feel different.

They might lose their hair.

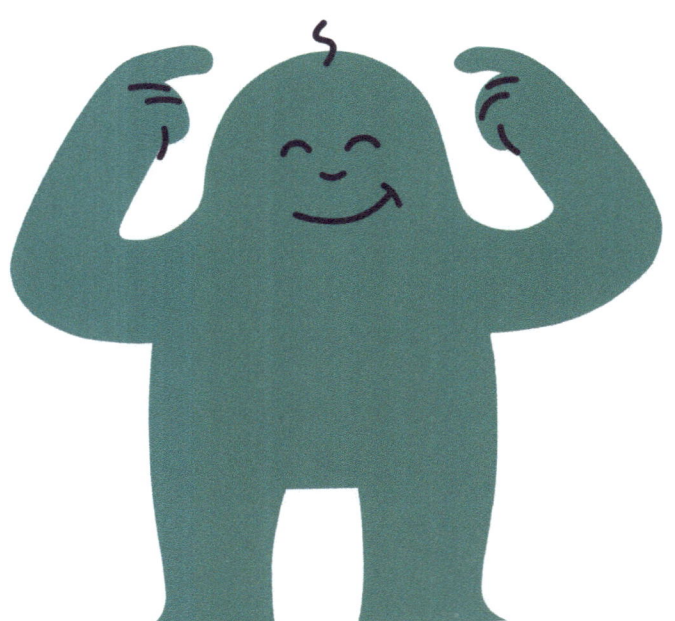

They might feel tired.

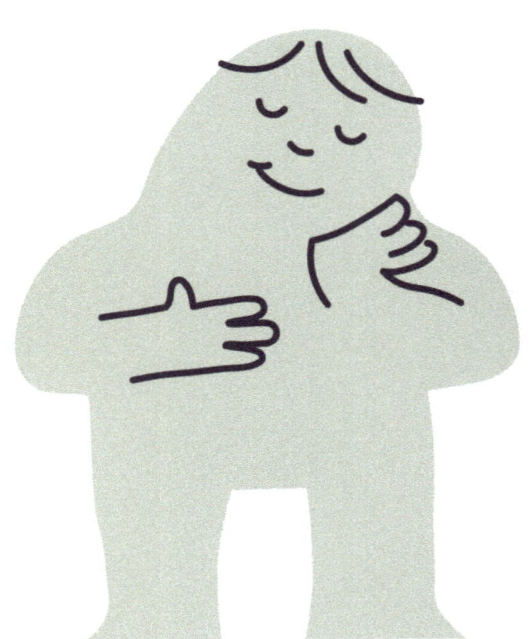

But doctors and nurses can give medicine to help them feel more comfortable.

And, sometimes they may like to play games, or watch their favorite movie, or snuggle a stuffed animal to help them feel comfortable.

Their stomach might feel upset.

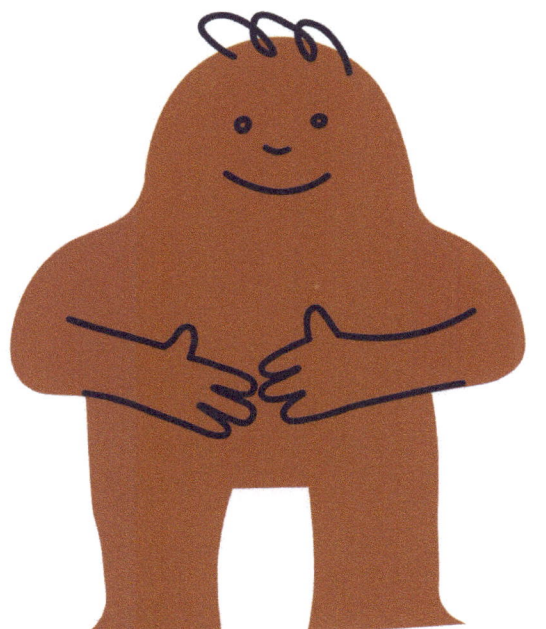

Their mouth and throat might feel yucky.

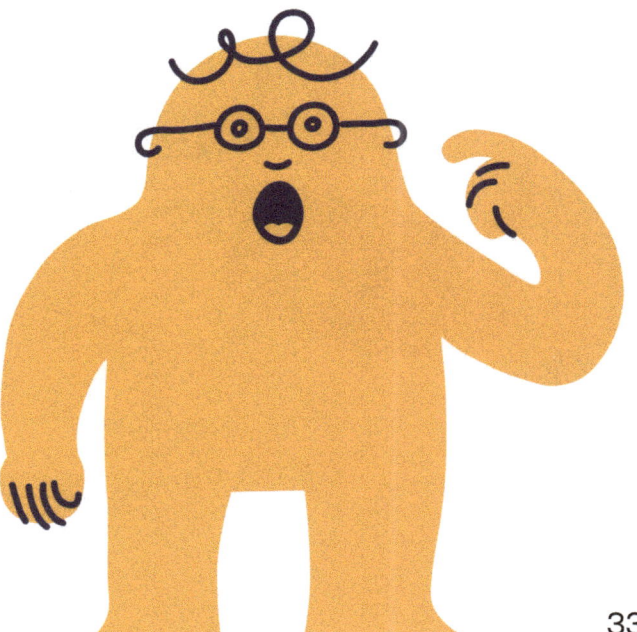

When someone is starting to feel better they will be able to...

eat and drink more of the foods they like,

take medicine by mouth, like they do at home,

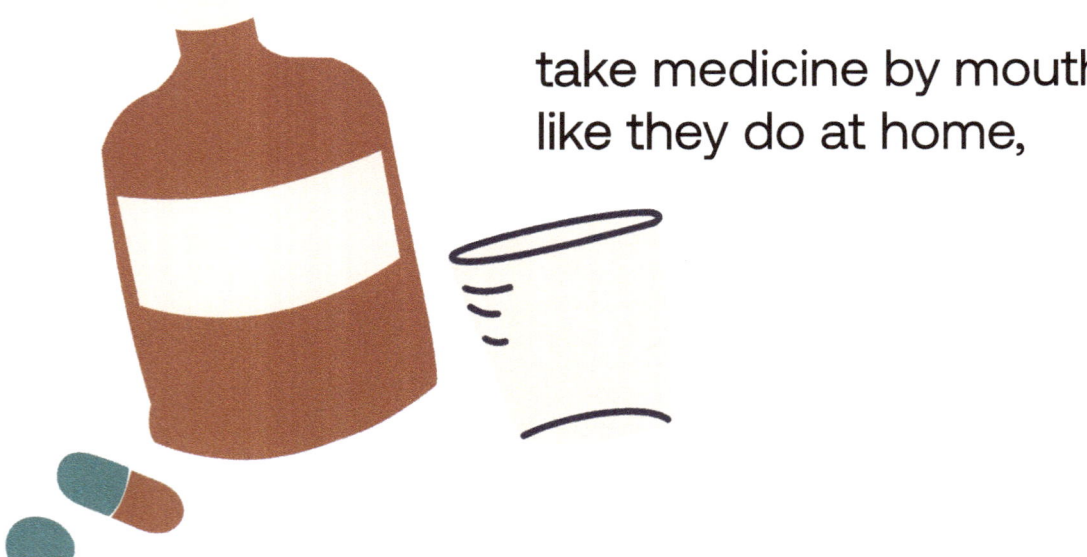

and have more energy to do their favorite activities.

When its time to go home, it will still be important to protect their body from germs, so...

a mask may need to be worn outside the house,

medicine may still be a part of their day at home,

and there may still be doctors visits to check on the healthy cells.

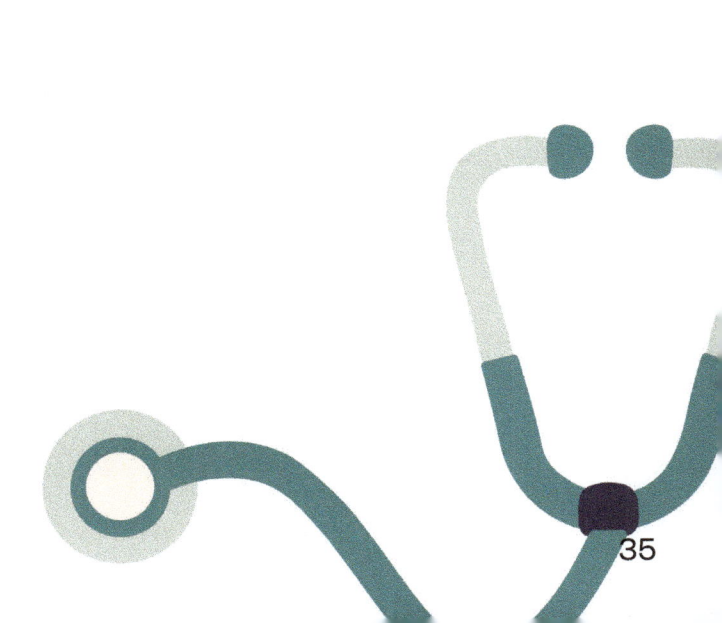

Now, we both know more about a bone marrow transplant. It is pretty amazing what our bodies can do!

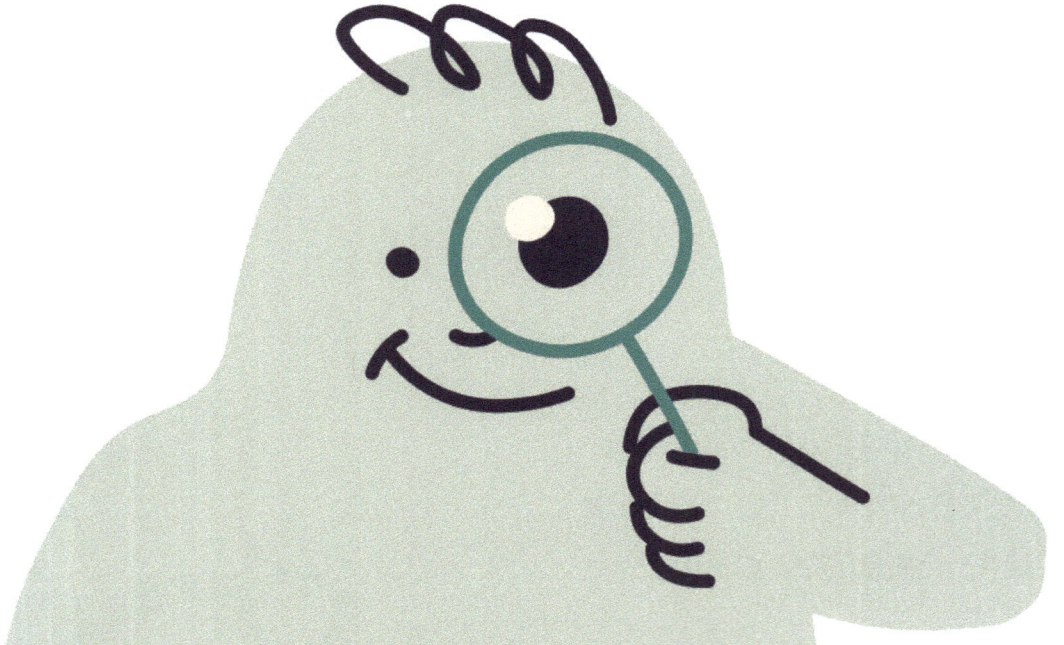

I wonder what I will learn about next!

Glossary

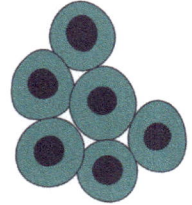

Cells:

Cells are tiny things that make up your body. They are so small you can't see them with your eyes, you need a microscope to see them. Every part of your body is made up of cells, both outside and inside. Your body also makes and replaces cells all the time. There are lots of different types of cells and they all have unique jobs that work together to keep your body strong and healthy.

Blood:

Blood is a system in your body that transports cells so they can do their jobs, it is kind of like a highway system.

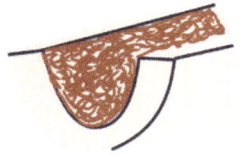

Bone Marrow:

Bone marrow is the squishy, middle part of your bones where blood is made, like a blood making factory. This is where baby blood cells, or stem cells, grow into adult blood cells.

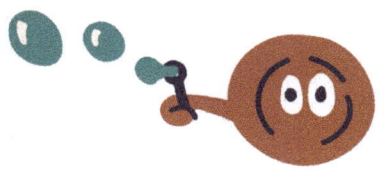

Red Blood Cells:

A type of cell that is found in your blood. Red blood cells carry nutrients, vitamins, and oxygen to your entire body, they also give you energy to run, jump, and play.

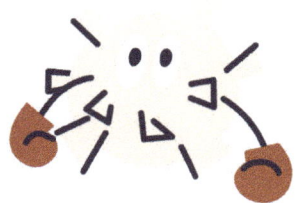

White Blood Cells:

A type of cell that is found in your blood. White blood cells help fight off germs or infections and help to keep you healthy.

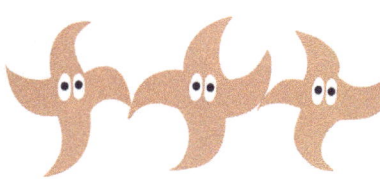

Platelets:

A type of cell that is found in your blood and helps your body heal. When your body gets hurt, platelets join together to form a seal to stop bleeding.

Do you know someone who needs a
bone marrow transplant?

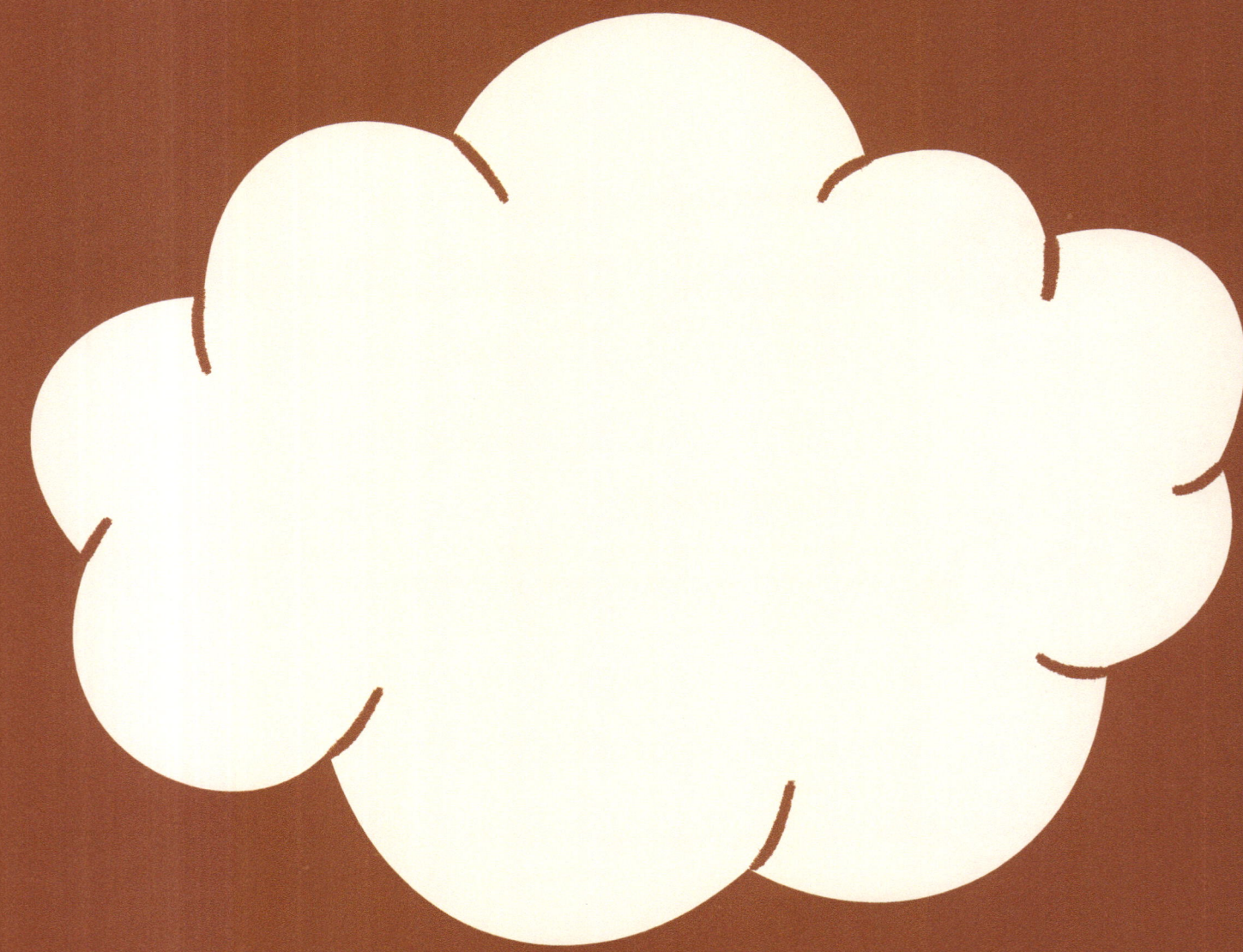

(talk about why someone you know may
be getting a bone marrow transplant)

Think of some activities that children could do in the hospital...

(draw activities you think of here)

I wonder what questions you might have?
Or, if you have questions later, who would you like to ask?

(draw a picture that could be hung up in the hospital while you think about your questions)

Color in the bone marrow filling back up with new, healthy bone marrow!

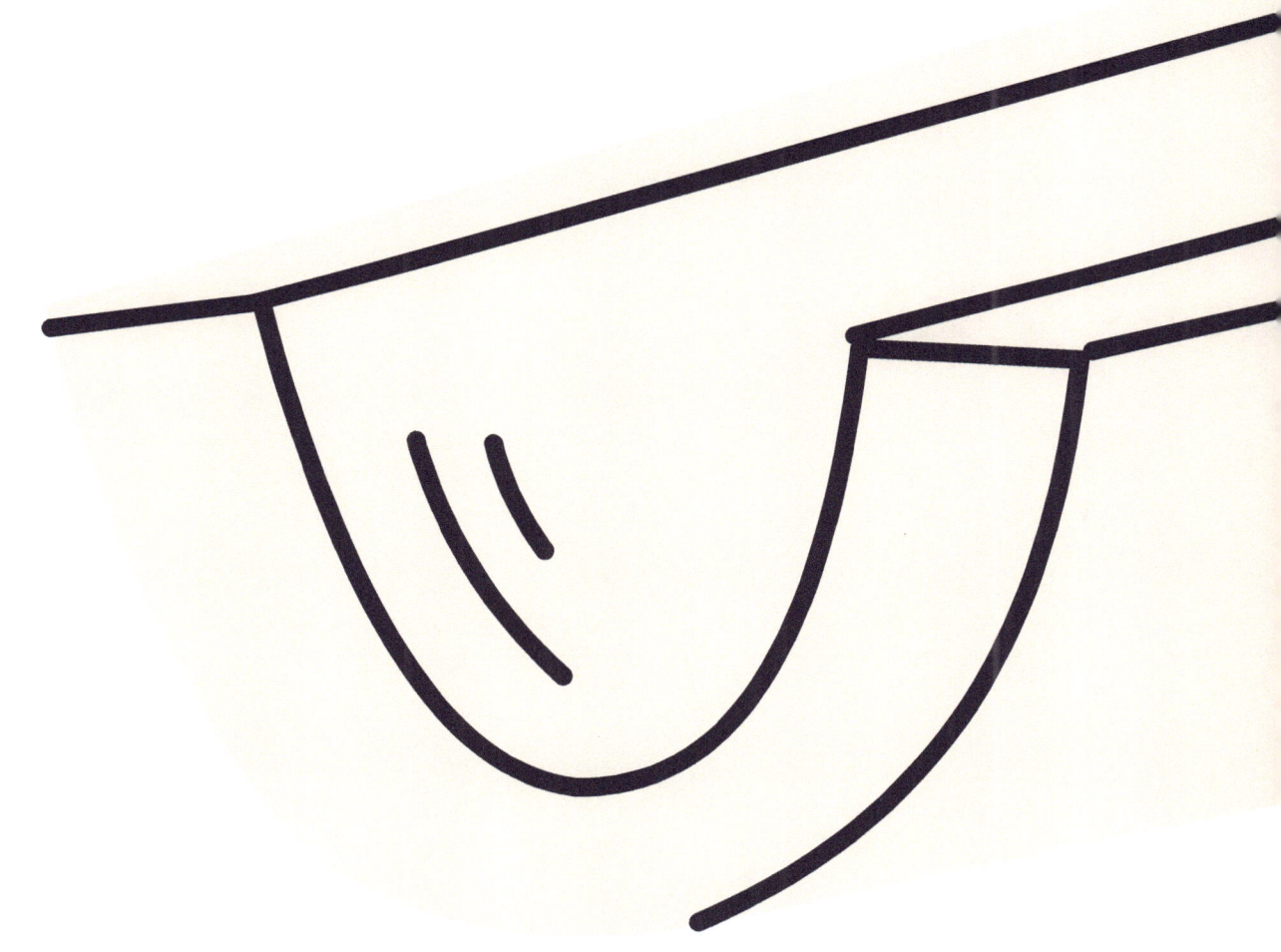

Conversation Tips for Talking to Your Child About a Bone Marrow Transplant (BMT)

How to begin talking to your child about why they, or someone they know, may need a bone marrow transplant (pg. 40)

This book can serve as the entry point into a tough conversation. With this book, at any point - before, during, or after - you can assess if the child has ever heard these words and if so, what do they understand about them.

Children understand their world in concrete terms. Identifying physical symptoms they themselves, or someone they know, have experienced or witnessed, helps them make sense of information. For example, is someone feeling more tired or unable to engage in activities they enjoy? Do they bruise more easily? Have they had to spend time in the hospital receiving medicine?

Relating physical symptoms back to the jobs of blood cells can help lead the conversation to the "why". A very general explanation could be, "someone needs a bone marrow transplant because their bone marrow, or blood making factory, isn't working how it is supposed to and needs help."

You can take it a step further, or have a future conversation, and address why the blood making factory is not working. Perhaps a child was born with a bone marrow system that did not work correctly, or their bone marrow has a difficult time making the correct cell shape needed to give them energy, or their body may not make enough blood cells to keep their body safe from germs

If you are having a difficult time finding the right words to explain the "why", please contact us at hello@childcorefamilysupport.com to receive some 1:1 support on how to talk to your child about a diagnosis.

Brainstorming activities to do in a hospital setting (pg. 41)

When someone is in the hospital, it can be helpful to have activities to focus on. This helps provide an element of distraction, brings a sense of familiarity or comfort, and can even facilitate development and healing. Some examples are, color a picture to hang up in a hospital room, read books, watch movies, play games/cards, or do puzzles.

If your child or child's sibling is the one who is anticipated to be in the hospital for an extended period of time, include them in the experience of packing the hospital bag.

If it is a peer or family member that is anticipated to be in the hospital for an extended period of time, this could be a time to help the child think of an toy/item, or letter, or picture they could send along with them.

Checking-in about any questions your child may have or things they are curious about (pg. 42)

Children are curious about the world around them. It is important to create opportunities for children to have space and feel comfortable asking questions or sharing what they are wondering about or worried about. This allows caregivers the chance to clarify any misconceptions (children have amazing imaginations), provide reassurance, and give information that is specific the individual child, thus, decreasing feelings of being overwhelmed with too much information.

You may be surprised at the things that are important to your child and thus, what their questions are. Some children need time to process information or they may need time to gather the courage to ask their questions. Therefore, check in with your child at various times following the book, this communicates to the child that the door is always open to talk to you and you are a safe space.

Scan the QR code to gain access to additional resources to help guide any adult through helping a child understand and cope with a bone marrow transplant.

Thank you to all of the Child Life Specialists
out there supporting children and their families!
We hope you hear it often,
but you are doing amazing work!

A personal thank you to Kim Ong for
providing such amazing guidance as a mentor and friend,
and Rose Tandeta for sharing her amazing expertise and edits!

Also to Brendan O'Connor for supporting our
efforts visually and helping us find our brand!

About the Authors

Child Core Family Support is a Child Life Specialist run company that provides consultation, resources, and information to caregivers of children going through medical experiences as well as support for providers who serve these families.

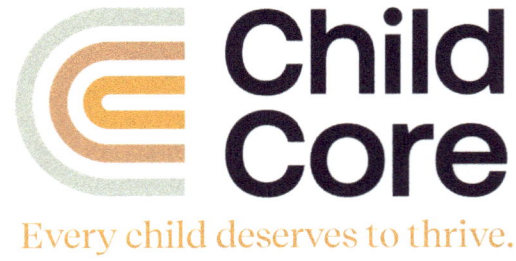

Their educational library strives to equip caregivers and professionals with the tools to feel confident and empowered when supporting a child through medical complexities. Child Core also offers free caregiver guides for talking to a child about a medical experience, and 1:1 coaching to meet the unique needs of individual families.

Find more information, resources, or to learn about child life specialists visit our WEBSITE.

www.ingramcontent.com/pod-product-compliance
Lightning Source LLC
Chambersburg PA
CBHW040005040426
42337CB00033B/5230